The Playdate
BUSY BOOK

The Playdate
BUSY BOOK

Heather Kempskie and Lisa Hanson

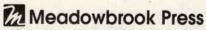

Meadowbrook Press
Distributed by Simon & Schuster
New York

Library of Congress Cataloging-in-Publication Data
     This title was previously cataloged with the following information:
Hanson, Lisa, 1973-
  The siblings' busy book : 200 fun activities for kids of different ages / by Lisa Hanson
and Heather Kempskie.
     p. cm.
  Includes index.
  ISBN 978-0-88166-530-7 (Meadowbrook Press),
  ISBN 978-0-684-05785-9 (Simon & Schuster)
  1. Amusements. 2. Games. 3. Creative activities and seat work. 4. Brothers and sisters.
I. Kempskie, Heather. II. Title.
  GV1203.H336 2008
  790.1'922--dc22

                              2008012286

Simon & Schuster ISBN 978-1-476-70142-4
Meadowbrook Press ISBN 978-0-88166-587-1

Editor: Alicia Ester
Copyeditor: Megan McGinnis, Liya Lev Oertel
Proofreaders: Angela Wiechmann, Doug McNair, and Paula Fleming
Production Manager: Paul Woods
Creative Director: Tamara JM Peterson
Cover Art: Dorothy Scott
Cover Photo: :Dejan Ristovsk
Interior Illustrations: Laurel Aiello

© 2013 by Heather Kempskie and Lisa Hanson

Published by: Meadowbrook Press
               6110 Blue Circle Drive, Suite 237
               Minnetonka, Minnesota 55343

www.meadowbrookpress.com

BOOK TRADE DISTRIBUTION by Simon and Schuster, a division of Simon and
Schuster, Inc., 1230 Avenue of the Americas, New York, New York 10020

17 16 15 14 13   10 9 8 7 6 5 4 3 2 1

Printed in the United States of America

Dedication

To our childhood friends with whom we spent endless hours in imaginary play: Thank you for the incredible memories and inspiration. And to the many playmates of our children, Kyle, Noah, Brooke, and Jake: Through you and with you, we get to continue on with the fun!

Acknowledgments

This is no secret: We love to have fun. And this experience has been just that. Thanks to the great team at Meadowbrook Press who made this project enjoyable from start to finish. To Bruce Lansky—for his gift of knowing what parents would love to see in a Busy Book. We're incredibly thankful that you called us again! To Liya Lev Oertel for her encouragement and for keeping us on track.

To our friends and family—Mom, Dad, and Amy—who cheered us on and to our nephew, Jack, who reminded us on a daily basis of the sweet, energetic play of a two-year-old. And of course, we thank our husbands, Matt and Kevin, and our children, Kyle, Noah, Brooke, and Jake. You guys make everything fun.

Contents

Introduction

As twins, there's not much we haven't done together. Growing up, we spent a lot of time with each other playing, attending school, and reaching milestones. We learned early on how to exchange ideas, compromise, be creative, and share good times.

Our childhood neighborhood was flush with kids. We'd spend the day drawing chalk houses, setting up pretend classrooms, or getting a few rounds of kickball started at the end of our dead-end street. We knew it was time to come home when the streetlights went out. We knew we could count on the fact that tomorrow would bring even more fun.

Playdates can offer that same kind of wonder. This creative generation of parents wouldn't dare let busy lives and sparsely populated neighborhoods get in the way of their children having fun and making friends. And thus, we believe, is how the idea of playdates was born: a special time for kids of all ages to get together, create, imagine, and celebrate holidays or other milestones as a group. Playdates offer an added bonus for parents too: They afford opportunities for us "older" folk to form parental alliances (the same type of alliances we formed in our childhood neighborhoods) and get in on some innocent and wild fun (the same type of fun we had as kids!).

Inside the pages of this book are some of our favorite, re-imagined games and activities of years past. We've mingled many of the activities with modern touches that were inspired by watching our own children play.

We started sharing our ideas with friends and family members who, like us, longed for group activities that were easy to do, required simple materials, and encouraged positive interactions among children. Their enthusiastic response to our suggestions prompted us to conclude that other parents and caregivers of multiple children might benefit from our ideas, too. That conclusion culminated into the book you're holding in your hands: *The Playdate Busy Book,* the newest addition to Meadowbrook Press's popular Busy Book line.

About This Book

You'll find over two hundred activities in this book, and each has been designed to engage multiple children of varying ages. The great news is that this book can be used when you've got a group of children of all ages or if you've just invited the toddler playgroup over. All the activities have been parent tested and child approved! We've organized the book into themed chapters so you can easily find ideas for fun play outdoors and out on the town, plus indoor activities for when the weather keeps you inside. We've also included ideas for creative movement and music, kitchen adventures, learning exploration, arts and crafts, pretend play, seasonal celebrations, and more. In addition, we offer fun and positive ways your playgroup can work together as a team and make their world a better place.

Here's what you'll find in each activity:
- An easy-to-reference grid listing the materials you'll need for all ages (Safety note: The grid indicates the items *you* will need—not necessarily the items that are safe for that age group to use themselves. For example, you may need scissors or glue to complete the activity *for* the baby—but do not give the scissors or glue *to* the baby.)
- A brief overview explaining setup and general instructions
- Developmentally appropriate guidelines for four separate age groups (Babies, Toddlers, Preschoolers, and School-Age Children)

Throughout the book, we've also included detailed illustrations, helpful host tips, and personal anecdotes about our own experiences enjoying these activities with our children.

Regardless of the ages of the children in your group, we suggest reading each activity in its entirety before getting started. This will not only give you the complete overview of the activity, but it will also allow you to tailor the activity to your playgroup's unique interests and abilities. Because children develop at different rates, you may find a suggestion for another age group will work better for a given child. For instance, in the activity "Strollin' through Nature" (page 120), a toddler may want to sort nature objects—the suggested activity for his age group—but he may also want to participate in the guessing game listed under instructions for preschoolers. This is a book that can grow with each child!

We also encourage you and your playgroup to be creative with each activity. Don't be afraid to modify it to better suit your play area, climate, or children's moods and interests.

Let the Playdate Fun Begin!

Writing this book together reminded us how special our own childhood friendships were. We realized that fun never has to end! Our hope for *The Playdate Busy Book* is that it'll help young children learn the beauty of friendship and the importance of having fun. If you have any questions or comments about this book, you can e-mail us or write us in care of Meadowbrook Press. We'd love to hear from you!

Heather Lisa

P.S. In recognition of that fact that kids do indeed come in two sexes, we alternate the use of masculine and feminine pronouns throughout this book.

Chapter 1

Rainy Day Fun

Learn to love rainy days. When it's pouring outside, linger in your pajamas longer, enjoy breakfast at a more leisurely pace, and claim the day as yours.

—Lisa

It's easy for kids to feel cooped up when it rains, but in this chapter, you'll find simple and fun activities to bring out the sunny side of bad weather! We've included our favorite indoor activities and games, like building with blocks and playing hide-and-seek, plus silly art projects and creative games that will get kids moving. There's even an indoor picnic. These activities may even have children wishing for rain!

Having a Rolling Ball

Here's a fun game sure to topple the rainy-day blues.

What You'll Need	All Ages	Babies	Toddlers	Preschoolers	School-Age Children
Empty plastic bottles (or disposable cups)	✋				
Brightly colored balls	✋				

Set up the plastic bottles to serve as bowling pins in a hallway or a large room with lots of open space. The children can roll the balls toward the pins to knock them down.

Babies

Babies older than six months can roll a ball toward the pins with some help. For an interactive activity, have one of the older children roll a ball slowly toward the baby. She may even be able to grab the ball and roll it back. Babies younger than six months may have fun just watching the other kids knock down bottles with colorful balls.

Toddlers

As toddlers grow, they will begin to explore their ability to manipulate objects. You or a school-age child can show a toddler how to bowl by spreading his legs and bending over to roll the ball "granny style" toward the bottles. Trying to knock down the bottles will challenge his hand-eye coordination—let him stand as close to the pins as he needs to!

Preschoolers

As preschoolers become better at controlling the direction of the ball, their ability to focus will intensify. Add another challenge to this activity: After a preschooler knocks down the bottles, have an older child retrieve the ball and roll it back for the preschooler to catch.

School-Age Children

Challenge school-age children by giving them a smaller ball to roll. They can keep track of the number of pins they knock over, then try to beat their record each time. They can also help reset the bottles after another child's turn. Suggest they set the pins up in different formations.

Host Tip

Kids are ready for sign language at about six months of age. To teach the sign for *ball*, hold your arms in front of you, hands apart as if holding a ball, then slowly bring your hands toward each other.

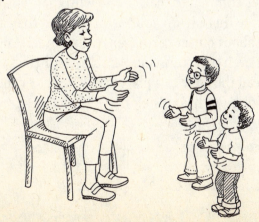

Hide-and-Seek Sounds

Sounds will help lead kids to their playmates in this hide-and-seek game.

What You'll Need	All Ages	Babies	Toddlers	Preschoolers	School-Age Children
Objects that make sounds, including spoons, musical toys, blocks, or bells	✋				

Have one child (the seeker) count to ten with his or her eyes closed while other children (the hiders) hide. You and/or an older child can partner up with any babies or toddlers. Each hider should have an item that makes a sound. To keep the hiding area manageable, have the kids hide in only a few adjoining rooms.

Babies

Instruct older children to make noise with their objects so the baby can locate them (with your help). During their first year, babies learn about object permanence, the understanding that objects exist even when unseen. Searching for the source of a sound will lead the baby to a playmate! The baby can also hide and create noise (with your help).

Toddlers

Like babies, toddlers may need help when it's their turn to
seek. This part of the game is a great opportunity to practice
counting to ten! Slowly count with the toddler and then say,
"Ready or not, here we come!" As a hider, a toddler will
discover how different objects can make different sounds—
loud or quiet, sharp or soft. While he waits to be found, the
anticipation will surely lead to giggles.

Preschoolers

Preschoolers will love seeking all by themselves. They'll probably find everyone rather quickly! As a hider, a preschooler may
find clever hiding places to keep the seeker guessing. Because
it's no fun to hide in one spot too long, expect a preschooler to
make plenty of noise to attract the seeker.

School-Age Children

When a school-age child is the seeker, he'll thrill the hiders if
he says something like, "I can't seem to find anyone. Where
did everybody go?" When it's his turn to hide, give him the
option to create sounds with his voice. Maybe he'll want to
sound like a beating drum or a hooting owl.

Shadow, Shadow on the Wall

Introducing the fun shadow show, starring kids' adorable hands and fingers!

What You'll Need	All Ages	Babies	Toddlers	Preschoolers	School-Age Children
Flashlight	🖐				
Black paper					🖐
Child-safe scissors					🖐

Grab a flashlight and dim the lights. Have the children face a wall and then shine the light in front of them. Let them follow the light as you make it dance across the wall and ceiling. Hold a hand in front of the light to cast a shadow on the wall and wiggle your fingers to create a spider shadow. Now it's the kids' turn to cast shadows. One of them can hold the flashlight steady as another casts a shadow.

Babies

The flashlight's bright light will transfix a baby as she develops her ability to visually track moving objects. If she is mobile, she may enjoy trying to catch the light. Point the flashlight toward the floor directly in front of her and move it slowly away as she tries to catch it.

Toddlers

For a fantastic cognitive exercise, a toddler can hold the flashlight. He will begin to recognize that the light moves when his hand does. When it's his turn to cast shadows, you or an older playmate can hold the flashlight for him. Encourage the toddler to wiggle his fingers to create a spider image. He can make his spider fast, slow, silly, or sleepy. Describing the spider is a great way to build his growing understanding of adjectives.

Preschoolers

Let preschoolers practice manipulating their fingers and hands any way they choose. Encourage them to use their imagination to describe their shadow inventions to playmates. For a fun guessing game, they can make animal sounds to accompany their shadow creations. Playmates can try to guess the animal. If a preschooler wants assistance, show her how to make a dog shadow: Have her press her palms together, bending her thumbs to create ears. She can move her ring and pinky fingers together to open and close the dog's mouth.

School-Age Children

With practice, a school-age child's shadows may be more sophisticated. He may even teach his playmates a few tricks! For even more fun, provide him with black paper and scissors. He can cut out small shapes in the paper, then hold the paper in front of the flashlight to cast more elaborate shadows. For instance, he can cut small holes to create a starry sky, or he can cut out a half-moon shape to create a peaceful night scene.

Host Tip

In addition to making shadow puppets, have kids move their bodies closer to and farther from the flashlight, making their shadows bigger and smaller.

Did You Know?

No one knows exactly when shadow puppetry began, but some historians estimate that prehistoric people practiced it as a way to express themselves or tell a story.

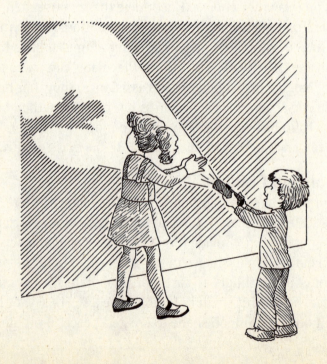

Hoop Ball Toss

Shoot baskets indoors with this fun tossing game.

What You'll Need	All Ages	Babies	Toddlers	Preschoolers	School-Age Children
Hula-Hoop	🖐				
Two couch cushions (or two chairs)	🖐				
Balls	🖐				

While the kids gather all the balls they can find, place two couch cushions on the floor and sandwich a Hula-Hoop upright between them. (You can also prop the hoop between two chairs.) Make sure there's enough space around the hoop and the cushions so the kids can get around them easily.

Babies

If the baby is crawling, encourage him to crawl through the hoop. Then kneel in front of the hoop with him and see if he can toss a small ball through it. If he's younger than six months, lay him on his back and gently roll a soft ball (a beach ball works well) over his tummy, legs, and arms. This action will help him become aware of his body parts.

Toddlers

When tossing the ball, a toddler can stand as close to the hoop as she'd like. Before she makes each toss, count a hearty "1-2-3!" to cheer her on. Station an older child on the other side of the hoop to retrieve and return the ball.

Preschoolers

This activity is a great opportunity to teach a preschooler different ways to toss a ball—overhead, underhand, sideways, and however else you like!

School-Age Children

If space allows, have a school-age child take two steps back each time she successfully tosses the ball through the hoop. She can start close to the hoop and, with skill, move back across the room. If the room is too small for this variation, see if she can toss the ball through the hoop with her eyes closed or while standing on one leg.

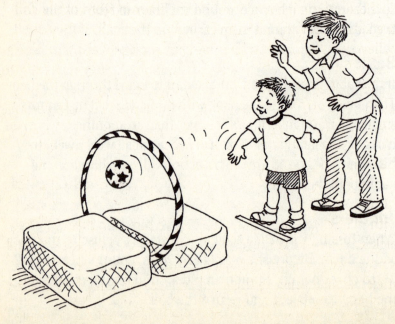

Jazzin' Up Junk Mail

Put your junk mail to good use with this creative and crazy activity.

What You'll Need	All Ages	Babies	Toddlers	Preschoolers	School-Age Children
Junk mail	🖐				
Tape	🖐				
12 x 12-inch sheets of clear contact paper	🖐				
Empty tissue box			🖐		
Pencil or marker					🖐

Gather junk mail and place it on the floor in front of the children. Announce that it's time to rip up the mail. If they don't believe you, show them by ripping up a piece! Let them have a blast tearing and crinkling up the junk mail. They may want to tape a sheet of clear contact paper sticky side up in front of them to make fun collages with the mail pieces. (Keep your eyes open for good coupons during this activity!)

Babies

Babies love to hear crinkling and tearing paper. If the baby can sit up and is at least six months old, he can rip up some mail with his playmates. (Make sure to give him thin pieces.) Then pick out some larger pieces, put the baby in his highchair, and tape contact paper onto the tray. With your help, let the baby stick the torn paper to the contact paper. He'll love feeling the sticky texture.

Toddlers

Toddlers simply may enjoy a chance to make a mess—never mind the art project. An empty tissue box will serve as the perfect mailbox where they can stuff junk-mail scraps. Let them empty and refill the box over and over again.

Preschoolers

Most preschoolers will be energetic when tearing up the mail, but may become contemplative when planning a collage. For a great motor-skill activity—and a new art technique—show them how to curl a strip of torn paper by wrapping it around a finger. You can also show them how to make waves or flames by making ragged tears along the edge of paper.

School-Age Children

Most pieces of junk mail are advertisements. To make a collage, school-age children can tear out images of products they or one of their playmates like (for example, a ball for baby, a stuffed animal for toddler, a toy car for preschooler, a coffee mug for Mom). They can then label the images with the playmates' names.

Host Tip

Have kids help you put the leftover junk-mail pieces into a large, heavy-duty plastic bag. Tie the bag shut, then encourage the children to roll, sit, or lie on the bag and listen to the crinkly noises it makes!

Crazy Sheet

Use a sheet to get kids moving, laughing, and working together.

What You'll Need	All Ages	Babies	Toddlers	Preschoolers	School-Age Children
One large sheet	🖐				
Plush animal	🖐				

Spread a large sheet on the floor of a room with lots of space and have the children gather around it. Play the following games for some crazy fun! (For most of these games, you'll need at least two players who are toddler age or older. For Parachute, you'll need four players.)

The Wave

Have the children kneel on the floor and each hold a corner of the sheet. Tell them to wave their arms dramatically to create movement. A baby can sit in your lap and wave his arms, too.

Popcorn

Instruct the children to hold the sheet close to the floor and quickly make little, low pops with it. If the baby can sit up, place him on the middle of the sheet. If not, lay him on the middle. He'll love watching the sheet "pop" up around him.

Parachute

Have the children hold the sheet close to the floor, then work together to raise it above their heads as quickly as possible. Then have them take a couple of steps forward while lowering the sheet behind them to turn the sheet into a parachute. Let a baby lie or sit underneath the sheet so she can watch it rise and fall around her.

Astronaut

Put an astronaut (a plush animal) on the middle of the sheet. Begin a countdown: "3-2-1, blastoff!" Raise the sheet up quickly to launch the astronaut into space. A baby may squeal in response to the blastoff and will anticipate the next one during the countdown.

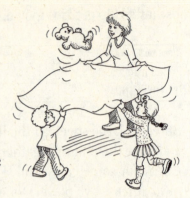

Spins

Hold on to the sheet and walk, jump, or skip in a circle. Hold the baby in your arms face out so she can see everyone's efforts to make the sheet spin.

We played these games when my parents were visiting. It was great having two extra pairs of hands. My son's favorite part was watching his beloved plush animal fly into the air during the astronaut game. He wanted to do it over and over again!

—Lisa

Build It Up!

Gather some budding builders and explore the fun of blocks!

What You'll Need	All Ages	Babies	Toddlers	Preschoolers	School-Age Children
Wood building blocks in all shapes and sizes	🖐				
Deck of cards					🖐

Place the wood blocks on a floor or table. These simple objects will provide developmental stimuli for every child, regardless of age.

Babies

Small wood blocks will be fun for a baby to hold and manipulate. Show her how to knock two blocks together to make noise. Babies six months or older may hold one block, see a second block, then drop the first one to retrieve the second.

Toddlers

Toddlers will enjoy learning how to balance, bridge, and brace the blocks to create a tower. They'll have fun knocking down the tower, too!

Preschoolers

By this age, preschoolers will begin to create more recognizable objects, like skyscrapers or other buildings. If the blocks have letters on them, encourage the kids to build towers that spell their names.

School-Age Children

In addition to the blocks, give school-age children a deck of playing cards. Show them how to use two blocks to sandwich a playing card. They can do this several times to make a fence. They can also make a roof by laying cards across parallel blocks. A steady table is a must!

Feather Frenzy

Get active with these fun feather games that teach patience, coordination, and teamwork.

What You'll Need	All Ages	Babies	Toddlers	Preschoolers	School-Age Children
Feathers (available at local craft store)	🖐				
Straws			🖐		
Medium-size hardcover books	🖐				

Feather Poem

Have each child hold a feather. As you recite the following poem, children can act out the movements it describes. You can assist a baby with this activity.

A feather on my hand (Place it on hand.)
A feather tickles my cheek (Touch it to cheek.)
A feather behind my back (Place it behind back.)
A feather under my feet (Brush the bottom of foot.)
A feather the tallest of all (Hold it up in the air.)
Now watch my feather fall (Release it.)

This poem encourages children to bend and stretch while coordinating words with movement.

Feather Blow

Have children lie on their bellies on the floor (an uncarpeted floor works best). Set a feather in front of each child. Encourage them to move their feathers across the floor by making an O shape with their mouths and blowing. To help a toddler direct his blowing, give him a straw to blow through. While older children race their feathers across the floor, hold a feather in front of a baby's face and gently blow on it. You can also brush it against his cheeks and hands. He will love the soft sensation.

Feather Race
Give each child a medium-size hardcover book. Stand near the children and drop a feather. Encourage the kids to work as a team to keep the feather in the air by waving their books like fans. This is a great workout for children's arms and a challenging hand-eye coordination activity. A baby can't help keep the feather aloft, but she'll enjoy waving her own book or will love feeling the cool breeze from her playmates' books.

Packin' a Picnic

When it's raining outside, create some sunshine inside by enjoying an indoor picnic.

What You'll Need	All Ages	Babies	Toddlers	Preschoolers	School-Age Children
Picnic snacks (see table on page 21)	🖐				
Blanket	🖐				
"Outdoor" items, such as plastic bugs, a picture of the sun, a houseplant, or flowers	🖐				
Paper plates, plastic utensils, and napkins	🖐				
Picnic basket or paper grocery bag	🖐				
Aluminum foil	🖐				

Older playmates can create a lovely picnic in a living room while you prepare the food. At the end of this activity you will find some examples of picnic snacks, but feel free to create your own menu!

Babies

If a baby is six months or older, sit him in a bouncy seat for the perfect view of the picnic. He'll still be perfecting his pincher grasp, so give him some plastic spoons to play with. If he's younger than six months, lay him on the picnic blanket close to an adult so he can see his playmates' faces and enjoy the scents of your food.

Toddlers and Preschoolers

Toddlers and preschoolers can spread out a blanket on the living room floor. With assistance, toddlers can straighten each corner. Then have them gather objects that remind them of the outdoors (for example, plastic bugs, a colored picture of the sun, a houseplant, or a vase of flowers) and place them around the blanket to create a more authentic-looking picnic scene.

School-Age Children

School-age children can place plates, utensils, and napkins on the blanket as well as help pack the picnic in a basket or grocery bag. Have them wrap the food in aluminum foil. They can play hosts by passing out the food after everyone is seated.

Host Tip

Help set the scene for the children. Tell them to imagine that it's a beautiful, sunny day, and you're outside for a picnic. What sounds do they hear? What things do they see? This exercise can help children for the rest of their lives. Visualization is a great tool for calming oneself in stressful situations.

Note: Be sure to ask about allergies any of the children may have before planning the snacks!

Picnic Snacks		
Snack	Age	Ingredients
Banana Bonanza	Babies six months or older	Mashed ripe bananas
Flower Bed	Toddlers, preschoolers, and school-age children	Crackers topped with hummus and sliced cucumber
Picnic Juice	Toddlers, preschoolers, and school-age children	Lemonade
Bug Bag	Toddlers, preschoolers, and school-age children	Sandwich bags filled with crackers, gummi worms, and raisins or other dried fruit (Make sure a toddler's bag has only pediatrician-approved foods and avoid those that could pose a choking hazard.)
Ants on a Log	Preschoolers and school-age children	Celery pieces topped with cream cheese (or peanut butter) and raisins

Collection Binders

Introduce children to collecting with this simple, inexpensive activity.

What You'll Need	All Ages	Babies	Toddlers	Preschoolers	School-Age Children
Computer with printer and Internet access (or magazines)	✋				
Three-ring binders	✋				
Printer paper	✋				
Three-holed sheet protectors	✋				
Child-safe scissors	✋				
Glue sticks	✋				
Collection items					✋
Pencil					✋

This activity is a great way to discover each child's interests. Children can collect images from their home computers or magazines for their collection binders, which they can add to again and again. If you print images from the computer, simply slip the pages into sheet protectors. When using magazine cutouts, glue them onto paper, allow them to dry, and slip them into the sheet protectors. Place each child's collection into separate binders.

Babies

For a baby's collection, ask playmates about what they think he loves. Possible items include a rattle, doll, blanket, or other small toy. Pick one item and work with children to find images on your computer or in magazines. Be sure to show each image to the baby while you describe it: For example, "This is a rattle." Slip the images into sheet protectors, then place them in a binder. Let the baby look through the pictures as often as possible with you and his playmates.

Toddlers

Let toddlers choose a particular toy, color, or character that's most special to them. Find images of their favorite things and let them point to the ones they want to add to their binder. After you cut out the images, they can glue them onto the paper. With assistance, they can then slide the paper into the sheet protectors and add the pages to their binder.

Preschoolers

A collection binder gives preschoolers the opportunity to use such skills as organizing, sorting, and categorizing. Help them decide what categories are in their collection. They could include animals, people, and flowers. Write each category on a separate sheet of paper, which the kids can use as dividers in their binder. Have them organize their images accordingly. They can bring their collection binder with them to school, to their grandparents' house, or to the park. They'll gain self-esteem by having something that reflects their unique interests.

School-Age Children

Perhaps the school-age children collect baseball and other cards, stickers, or toy cars. Invite them to set up a display of these items for their playmates to view. They can write descriptions or include photos or images of their collection in their binder, creating an inventory of their items.

Host Tip
The Internet can be a wonderful resource when used properly. Take time to review Internet safety with the children and always supervise while they use the computer.

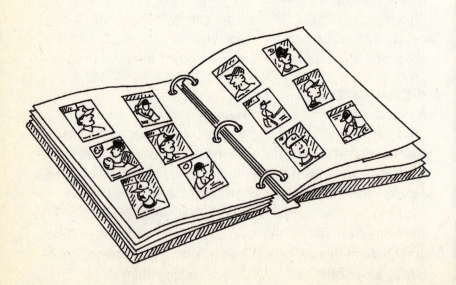

It's a Wrap

In this activity, children will discover it's just as fun to wrap objects as it is to unwrap them.

What You'll Need	All Ages	Babies	Toddlers	Preschoolers	School-Age Children
Gift-wrap	✋		✋	✋	
Boxes of various sizes			✋	✋	✋
Objects to wrap (books, small toys, and so on)			✋	✋	✋
Toy blocks		✋			
Child-safe scissors			✋	✋	✋
Tape			✋	✋	✋
Stickers			✋		
Crayons			✋		

Break out gift-wrap and different-size boxes, and let playmates wrap up objects for fun. When they're done, have them exchange "gifts" and enjoy undoing their handiwork.

Babies

If the babies are older than six months, lay some gift-wrap over a few toy blocks for them to "unwrap." Whether the babies are sitting in a highchair or crawling toward the hidden blocks on the floor, this hide-and-seek game will have them using their motor skills to grab and hold the paper. For babies younger than six months, hold a piece of brightly colored gift-wrap in front of them and slowly begin to crumple it. Hide it behind your back and crumple it again. Playfully ask, "Where did that noise come from?"

Toddlers

Give toddlers empty boxes and invite them to place an object, like a book or small toy, in each box as a pretend gift. Because wrapping the gift may be difficult at this age, cut shapes from the gift-wrap and help toddlers tape them to the box. Also provide toddlers with some stickers and crayons to decorate their boxes.

Preschoolers

Help preschoolers measure and cut the appropriate amount of gift-wrap. Show them how to fold the paper to cover the box, and stick pieces of tape to the edge of the table so the kids can easily retrieve them. Grabbing and placing the tape is an excellent motor-skill exercise.

School-Age Children

Cutting gift-wrap and wrapping gifts are great ways for school-age children to learn how to estimate, measure, and solve problems. Have them each secretly wrap an object and then provide clues for each other as they try to guess what it is.

The Home Highway

Rev up your engines—it's time for an indoor highway game that will get kids moving!

What You'll Need	All Ages	Babies	Toddlers	Preschoolers	School-Age Children
Child-safe scissors	✋				
Red, yellow, green, and white construction paper	✋				
Markers	✋				
Tape	✋				
Stroller		✋			
Toy car			✋		

To begin, you and any older children can create traffic signs for the highway. You can include traffic lights (green, red, and yellow), stop signs, railroad-crossing signs, one-way signs, and signs with arrows pointing left, right, or straight ahead. The kids can cut out the signs' shapes from the appropriate colors of construction paper (for example, an octagon from red paper) and add words and features with markers (for example, the word *STOP*). They can then tape the signs at eye level around the space to transform it into an active and busy street. Once the highway is complete, it's time for everyone to go for a "drive"!

Babies

Transport babies in strollers or hold them as you zoom around. Make car noises as you travel, including screeching brakes. At any age, babies will love moving quickly and hearing enthusiastic sounds!

Toddlers

Toddlers can bring a toy car along with them or they can be the cars. Point out the signs and teach them what they mean. For instance, "This big red sign says 'Stop.'" Say the word as you show the action. They may enjoy following the signs or making up their own rules.

Preschoolers and School-Age Children

Preschoolers and school-age children can help younger playmates by serving as friendly traffic cops. Show them how to signal *stop* (palm out, fingers upward), *go* (palm inward and motioning forward), and *turn left* or *turn right* (point in the correct direction).

Host Tip

This activity is a great opportunity to review street-crossing safety. Stand with the children on one side of the pretend highway and tell them to look both ways for cars. If they don't see any, it is safe to cross the street while holding a grownup's hand.

> I created a stop sign to put on the TV screen in our home. When the sign was up, my kids knew TV wasn't an option.
>
> —Heather

Indoor Scavenger Hunt

Playmates will need determination and sleuthing skills for this indoor scavenger hunt!

What You'll Need	All Ages	Babies	Toddlers	Preschoolers	School-Age Children
Index cards	🖐				
Markers	🖐				

For each playmate, use markers to create three age-appropriate visual clues (drawings of objects in the home) or verbal clues (words about objects in the home) on index cards. Give the clue cards to the children, and let the scavenger hunt begin!

Babies

A baby can enjoy the hunt, too, by crawling after playmates or riding in someone's arms. After each item is found, show the baby the image on the index card and then the corresponding object.

Toddlers

Give toddlers one card at a time, and give them additional hints about the objects' locations. Use prepositions to describe the items' locations, like *in*, *under*, *above*, *between*, and *below*, such as, "This object is under the coffee table."

Preschoolers

Preschoolers can use clue cards with drawings or, instead, receive verbal clues only, such as, "Find something you can build with that is square." This requires them to use creativity and deduction. They may find a block, a box, or anything else that fits the description.

School-Age Children

School-age children will be up for more of a challenge, so send them off to find several objects for each clue. Their clue cards should provide challenges such as, "Find three things in the house that hold things together." They may return with some tape, a bottle of glue, and a piece of string. Another example could include, "Find three things that are each spelled with two vowels." They may return with a book, banana, and shoe.

Host Tip

After the hunt is done, create another game to put the items away. For each item, challenge playmates to return it to its proper place by the time you (or an older child) count to ten.

Where Is the Boat?

There's essentially no setup and tons of guessing fun in this game!

What You'll Need	All Ages	Babies	Toddlers	Preschoolers	School-Age Children
Toy boat	🖑				

Playmates take turns being the "sailor," who stands with eyes closed facing away from the others. Hand a toy boat to one of the players and tell the child to quietly hide it. (The hiding place will depend on the sailor's age—see below. You may need to help the hider find an appropriate place for each sailor.) When the toy boat is hidden, the sailor opens his eyes and everyone chants:

Ahoy, [name of sailor]!
Your boat is lost at sea.
Wherever could it be?

The sailor then searches for the boat. If the sailor finds it, whoever hid the boat becomes the sailor. If the sailor doesn't find the boat, he remains the sailor for another turn.

Babies

When it is a baby's turn to be the sailor, have an older child hide the boat behind his or her back while you face the other direction with the baby. After the boat is hidden, hold the baby in front of each player for a few seconds as she contemplates which playmate has the boat. Babies will love looking at their playmates' expressive faces. When the baby reaches the hider, have the playmate dramatically reveal the boat and say, "Peekaboo!"

Toddlers

When it's a toddler's turn as sailor, make sure the other children know they must hide the boat somewhere in plain or partial view. Toddlers will love this game's suspense and will enjoy searching for the boat's location.

Preschoolers

Encourage the hider to place the boat somewhere out of sight when it's a preschooler's turn as sailor. To make it more fun, play "hot and cold" while a preschooler is searching. Say, "Cold," when he's far from the toy and, "Hot," when he gets closer to finding it.

School-Age Children

When it's a school-age child's turn, hide the boat completely out of sight. To challenge them, give school-age children a time limit, such as ten seconds, to find the boat.

Sharing a Smile

Just try to keep a serious face during this happy circle game!

What You'll Need	All Ages	Babies	Toddlers	Preschoolers	School-Age Children
Smiles!	✋				

Have playmates sit in a circle. The oldest child can start the game by smiling widely or making a funny face. His playmates must try their hardest not to smile in response. He can then use his hand to "wipe" the smile off his face, then "toss" it to one of his playmates, who then takes a turn smiling. The round ends after everyone has had a turn tossing a smile… or once everyone has started giggling. How long can they keep the round going?

Babies

Babies love faces. If a playmate tosses a smile to a baby, see if she can make a grin appear on the baby's face with a silly movement or sound.

Toddlers

Most toddlers mimic the emotions of others. If a toddler sees smiling faces all around him, he may join in. Have fun showing him how to wipe a smile off his face and how to throw it. If he smiles throughout the whole game, let him!

Preschoolers and School-Age Children
Preschoolers and school-age children are more able to control their facial expressions, so they may be champions at this game. Instead of tossing a smile, older children may pretend to hide it under their shirt, sit on it, or pull it through their ears in an attempt to make their playmates laugh!

Puzzle Making

Take out some puzzles or create your own on a rainy afternoon!

What You'll Need	All Ages	Babies	Toddlers	Preschoolers	School-Age Children
Plastic balls and wooden blocks		🖐			
Shoebox with lid		🖐			
Pencil		🖐			
Scissors		🖐	🖐	🖐	🖐
Puzzle with large pieces		🖐	🖐		
Empty cereal boxes			🖐	🖐	🖐
Crayons				🖐	🖐
Child-safe scissors				🖐	🖐

Babies

Babies six months or older can work on a homemade puzzle that's perfect for their age: a shape sorter. Gather some wooden blocks and plastic balls. On a shoebox lid, trace circles and squares big enough for the balls and blocks to fit through, then cut out the shapes. Place the lid back on the shoebox and encourage babies to slip the balls and blocks through the circles and squares. When they have dropped all the objects into the box, empty it out so they can repeat the fun!

For younger babies, help them explore the odd shapes of puzzle pieces. Run their fingers along the contours of a large, chunky puzzle piece—down the curves and over the bumps.

Toddlers

Place some puzzles with large, chunky pieces on the floor
for toddlers to put together. You can also create a homemade
puzzle: Cut the front of a cereal box into large pieces.
Toddlers can work to reassemble the familiar image.

Preschoolers and School-Age Children

Cut off the front and back of a cereal box and give one side to
each child. Have the kids decorate the back of the cardboard
with crayons. Suggest they draw large, realistic pictures of
people, vehicles, or houses. They can cut the cardboard into
large, chunky pieces. Then they can mix up the pieces and try
to put their puzzles back together again.

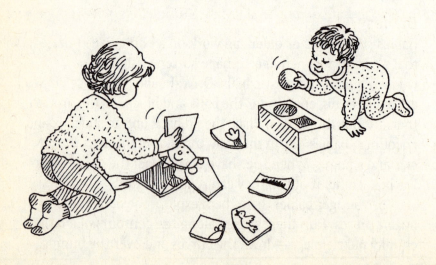

Terrific Tunnels

Turn any room into a twisty roadway complete with tunnels!

What You'll Need	All Ages	Babies	Toddlers	Preschoolers	School-Age Children
Large paper bags	✋				
Scissors	✋				
Masking tape	✋				
Toy trucks and cars			✋	✋	✋
Crayons				✋	
Books					✋
Blankets					✋
Chairs					✋

Cut out the bottoms of several paper bags. Tape the bottomless bags together end to end to create a tunnel. For wider tunnels, cut each bag along a crease, then tape two bags together where you cut. Tape your double-wide bags end to end to complete the tunnel.

Babies

For babies who are on the move and ready to explore, cruising in the tunnels will be a new experience. If they are younger than six months or not crawling yet, lay the babies on their tummies to look through a short tunnel. Have playmates look through the other end and play peekaboo.

Toddlers

Toddlers may get right to work crawling through the tunnels! Taking a toy truck with them will make the journey even more exciting. This pretend play is how toddlers begin to make sense out of things they see, like roads and cars.

Preschoolers

To get through the small tunnels, preschoolers may have to army crawl (pull themselves forward with their arms while dragging their legs behind them), which is great for building muscles and coordination in the upper half of their bodies. On their way through, they may stop to create roadways with crayons for toy cars for subsequent trips through the tunnels.

School-Age Children

School-age children can create cool ramps for toy cars by propping up one end of a tunnel with some books. They can place two toy cars at the top of the tunnel and see which car goes through the tunnel the farthest or the quickest. They can also use blankets draped over chairs to make tunnels of their own to crawl through. Or they may find a tunnel to be a quiet place to read a book, alone or with playmates.

Designer Dress Up

Let the kids be fashion designers!

What You'll Need	All Ages	Baby	Toddler	Preschooler	School-Age Child
Child-safe scissors			🖐	🖐	🖐
Scissors			🖐	🖐	🖐
Cardstock			🖐	🖐	🖐
Crayons			🖐	🖐	🖐
Glue sticks			🖐	🖐	🖐
Construction paper			🖐	🖐	🖐
Plush animal		🖐			
Baby clothes		🖐			

Cut small shirts, pants, skirts, hats, and shoes out of cardstock.
After you've cut a few pieces, encourage the children to be fashion
designers and color the clothes while you continue to cut more.
You may also want any toddlers and preschoolers to use their
cutouts as patterns to cut clothes of their own. When all the
clothing is cut out and colored, have children assemble entire
outfits and glue them to construction paper. If they want, they
can complete their pictures by filling in bodies and heads.

Babies

While older children work on their projects, this is the perfect
opportunity to teach babies about clothing. Do they have a
favorite plush animal? Sit close to them and let babies watch you
dress their favorite friend using baby clothes (a onesie, socks, or

shirt). Be sure to name each item you put on their friend. When you're done, sing a funny American folk song called "Down by the Bay." In the last line, describe the baby's friend:

> *Down by the bay, where the watermelons grow,*
> *Back to my home I dare not go.*
> *For if I do, my mother will say...*
> *"Have you ever seen a [duck wearing a shirt]*
> *down by the bay?"*

Toddlers

Give toddlers a few clothing cutouts and draw a person on their construction paper. To get them started, say, "This person needs shoes. Can you find a shoe for him?" Let them gaze over their choices and applaud their efforts when they point to a shoe. Let them show you where to glue it on the figure.

Preschoolers

Preschoolers will enjoy "designing" colorful garb for a trip to the beach or a fancy party. At this age, they know where each item should go when it's time to glue their outfit to construction paper. Their sense of humor may get the best of them, though: The shoes could end up coming out of shirt sleeves!

School-Age Children

After gluing their outfit onto construction paper, encourage school-age children to finish the scene by drawing a body and a backdrop. Ask them where their person might go in that outfit. For example, if they chose blue jeans and a T-shirt, they might draw a classroom or park in the background.

At the Movies

Rainy weather is the perfect excuse to cuddle with friends and enjoy a short movie.

What You'll Need	All Ages	Babies	Toddlers	Preschoolers	School-Age Children
Age-appropriate movie			🖐	🖐	🖐
Pillows and blankets	🖐				
Snacks (see suggestions below)			🖐	🖐	🖐
Construction paper and crayons			🖐	🖐	🖐

Make watching a movie a special event by putting soft pillows and blankets on the floor and darkening the room. See the "In the Kitchen" chapter for our favorite movie-time treats: "Toasted Banana Treat" (page 353), "Fragrant Cinnamon Buns" (page 354), and "Pizza Faces" (page 349).

Babies
The American Academy of Pediatrics recommends no TV for children under the age of two, so use your discretion if including a baby in this activity. We suggest you use this time to feed him or cuddle him while he rests.

Toddlers, Preschoolers, and School-Age Children
Make up some fun rules for your viewing time. For instance, whenever a song begins, everyone has to get up and dance. Or

if there's a bird in the movie, everyone has to pretend to fly. When the movie is done, try these fun activities:

- Discuss your favorite scenes and characters.
- Pass out construction paper and crayons, and ask the children to each draw their favorite scene.
- Re-create a scene by narrating it and having children act it out. There may be future actors in the crowd!

Host Tip

Preview a kid-friendly movie or get a recommendation by visiting an online source like Yahoo! Movies—Family Movies (http://movies.yahoo.com/family/).

Chapter 2

Let's Pretend

A dear friend of mine once told me about her five-year-old daughter's pretend play with future careers. The little girl had pretended to be a marine biologist—who was also a Mary Kay lady. She just had one question: "Can I have a day off?"

"Of course," her mom replied. "Most people have weekends off."

"Good," she said as she skipped out of the room. "That means I'll be a mermaid on weekends!"

—Heather

Is there anything as strong as a child's imagination? All children love pretend play, and they usually find it most enjoyable when others join them, which makes it the perfect pastime for playdate fun. In this chapter, we offer imagination-boosting activities that use simple props found in most homes. With special instructions to stimulate each age range in your group, kids will become astronauts, hairstylists, and doctors right before your eyes!

Check-Us-Out Library

Nurture children's love of reading by setting up a library.

What You'll Need	All Ages	Babies	Toddlers	Preschoolers	School-Age Children
Books	✋				
Index cards or slips of paper	✋				
Post-it Notes			✋		
Stamp and ink pad				✋	

Have the children gather a variety of books to create their library. They can display the books on tables, chairs, shelves, or the floor. Set up a checkout station and give each patron an index card or slip of paper as a library card.

Babies

The baby can be the first patron of this special library. Select a brightly illustrated board book for her to handle and mouth. Read the story to her or invite an older child to read it to everyone. The baby will associate reading with special time with you and her playmates.

Toddlers

Toddlers can help place a Post-it Note checkout card inside the front cover of every book, but they'll enjoy being a library patron more. Maybe they will find a new favorite book or recognize one they love from their own home (don't be surprised if they select an old favorite when it's their turn to check out books).

Preschoolers

Let preschoolers play the librarian. Set up a checkout station. They can use a stamp and ink pad to mark "Due Dates" on the checkout cards. They can also help patrons select books. Say to them, "I feel like reading a funny book. Can you select one for me, Mr. Librarian?"

School-Age Children

School-age children can decide how to display and organize the books in the library. For example, do they want to group the books by age range? Topic? Alphabetically by author or title? When they are done, have them give other patrons a tour of the library.

Mail for You and Me

Send and deliver mail right in your own home!

What You'll Need	All Ages	Babies	Toddlers	Preschoolers	School-Age Children
Paper grocery bag	🖐				
Scissors	🖐				
Paper cups		🖐			
Crayon			🖐		
Index cards			🖐	🖐	🖐
Large purse or lunch bag		🖐			
Envelopes				🖐	🖐
Stickers				🖐	
Pencil					🖐

To create a mailbox, close the top of a paper grocery bag, then fold it over and staple it shut. Cut a six-inch-by-two-inch slot in the front of the bag. Children can then get busy writing, sending, and delivering their letters.

Babies

Sing this twist on Woody Guthrie's "Mail Myself to You" with older kids while taking turns doing the following actions with the baby:

I am going to fold you up like an envelope. (Fold his arms gently with your hands.)
Put glue on your nose—you will see. (Gently tap his nose.)

Put stamps upon your head. (Gently tap his head.)
And mail you straight to me! (Hug him.)

If the baby is six months or older, he also may enjoy dropping his own "mail" into the mailbox. To create something easy for him to hold and thin enough to fit through the slot, cut the bottoms from a few paper cups. The small circles will be the perfect size.

Toddlers
Draw different shapes with a crayon on separate index cards and give them to the toddler. She can deliver these pretend postcards. For example, ask her to deliver the card with a circle to the baby or place the card with the square in the mailbox. She can even use her own mailbag (a purse or lunch bag) to make her deliveries.

Preschooler
Give preschoolers the supplies needed to send letters. They can stuff index cards into envelopes, put "stamps" (stickers) on the envelopes, and put the envelopes into the mailbox. Later, they can pretend to be letter carriers and deliver the mail to their playmates.

School-Age Children
Let school-age children gather the mail from the mailbox and prepare it for delivery. They can decide where each letter should be mailed by writing the name and address of a family member or friend on each envelope. Here's an opportunity for

them to memorize their own addresses: Have them write a return address on the top-left corner of every envelope.

Host Tip

This is a great time for school-age children to find a pen pal. The pen pal can be a cousin, aunt, or friend from school. Writing and receiving letters gives children self-confidence and a sense of belonging. It's also a wonderful way to learn the importance of language, writing, and communication skills. Have school-age children initiate the exchange by writing a letter to a person of their choice. They can write about school, hobbies, or a recent vacation. Encourage them to ask about the recipient's interests. Finally, teach them how to properly address an envelope and affix postage. With some help, even preschoolers can send a letter to a pen pal.

> My preschooler loves to receive mail, so we decided to send a letter to his cousin who lives a few hours away. My sister-in-law and I had to help write the boys' letters. The pen pals learned each other's favorite colors, what candy they like, and that they both loved superheroes. My son was thrilled each time a letter arrived.
>
> —Heather

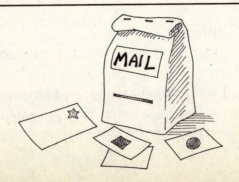

Toy Store Sale

Make the toys in your home seem brand-new by setting up a pretend toy store.

What You'll Need	All Ages	Babies	Toddlers	Preschoolers	School-Age Children
Toys	🖐				
Play money			🖐	🖐	🖐
Paper grocery bags			🖐		
Post-it Notes				🖐	
Crayons				🖐	
Shoebox or muffin pan					🖐

Have children each find a few toys to "sell," then help them create a toy store in a room in your home. Give each child some play money, and let them choose the toys they wish to buy!

Babies

Assign a playmate to select a few items just right for the baby and demonstrate to him how they work. For instance, a child may race a toy car in front of the baby. The baby will love the interaction and may try to imitate his friend at play. He will also love to hold, examine, and play with the toys picked especially for him.

Toddlers

Toddlers love to load and unload objects, making them the perfect people to stock the toy store! They can place toys on tables or couches and help load paper bags with merchandise.

To sharpen their listening skills and build their language skills, pretend to be a shopper and ask for "big" or "noisy" toys. They will try to identify the toys that meet your requests.

Preschoolers

Give preschoolers Post-it Notes to place on each toy. On them, they can write how much each toy costs. Have them use denominations that match the play money. Help them decide the cost of each toy based on its size and how fancy it is. This activity is a wonderful way to practice number recognition and introduce children to the value of money.

School-Age Children

This activity is perfect for strengthening school-age children's math skills. They can use a shoebox or muffin pan as a cash register, then collect the money and make change when someone makes a purchase.

Camping In

You don't have to be outdoors to enjoy this campsite!

What You'll Need	All Ages	Babies	Toddlers	Preschoolers	School-Age Children
Metal pots and pans	🖐				
Wooden spoon	🖐				
Bells		🖐			
Toy blocks	🖐				
Red and yellow tissue paper	🖐				
Blankets and pillows	🖐				
Large sheet (or chairs and rope or a real tent)	🖐				

Setting up camp is a big part of the fun. Children can help with the setup before enjoying the camping activities listed on the next page.

Babies

As older children set up camp, the baby can keep "wild animals" at bay. If she's old enough to sit up by herself, give her a metal pot and a wooden spoon and let her bang away. Or give her a bell to jingle. If she is younger, jingle the bell in front of her. She'll enjoy the tinkling sound.

Toddlers

With help, toddlers can create a pretend campfire. They can arrange toy blocks in a circle and place crumpled red and yellow tissue paper in the center of the circle.

Preschoolers

Preschoolers can do a number of tasks around camp. They can gather pots and pans for a pretend cookout. Once the tent is pitched, they can arrange the blankets and pillows inside it.

School-Age Children

To create a tent, school-age children can drape a large sheet over a table or set up two chairs, tie a rope between them, and drape a blanket over the rope. Or, if possible, you can help them set up a real tent.

Host Tip

Here are some creative ways to enjoy the campsite together:

- Read stories around a pretend campfire (or a real fireplace if you have one).
- Prepare a pretend meal of hot dogs and baked beans.
- Create the sound of a thunderstorm by gently drumming your fingers on a hardcover book, then gradually drumming harder. The children can lend their voices to create booming thunder.
- Sing campfire classics like "Do Your Ears Hang Low?" or "Clementine."
- Hike the area around your campsite.
- Fish in a make-believe lake (a blue blanket or sheet spread on the floor).
- Search for wildlife. Hide a few plush animals under chairs or tables and have the children search for them.

Barnyard Fun

Little farmers will love creating their own barn for their plush and plastic animals.

What You'll Need	All Ages	Babies	Toddlers	Preschoolers	School-Age Children
Blanket	👋				
Plush and plastic farm animals	👋				
Indoor riding toy			👋		
Buckets or plastic bowls			👋		
Brush			👋		
Hobbyhorse or large stick				👋	

Use a blanket draped over chairs to create an indoor barn. Let children complete the scene with plush or plastic farm animals.

Babies

Babies often learn and repeat one-syllable words before learning more complicated ones. This activity may encourage the baby to make an animal sound, perhaps as a first word! Sit in front of the baby and repeat an animal sound like "moo" or "oink" while slowly exaggerating your lip movements. See if he will repeat the sound. To help him associate objects with sounds, hold up a plush animal while making the appropriate sound.

Toddlers

If you have an indoor riding toy, have a toddler use it as a trac-tor around the barnyard. She can deliver toy buckets or plastic bowls filled with imaginary hay or feed for the animals. Give the toddler a small brush to groom the animals.

Preschoolers

Give preschoolers some riding lessons with a hobbyhorse (or a large stick). Show them how to straddle the horse and ride around the barn. To challenge their motor skills, have them walk, trot, and gallop their horses.

School-Age Children

School-age children can design a sign with a name for the barn. They also can name the farm animals and create signs for them to display inside the barn.

Host Tip

If you have a large appliance box, use that to create a barn. Draw and cut out barn doors that swing open and cut two squares for windows. Together, you and older children can paint the box red. Let it dry before using.

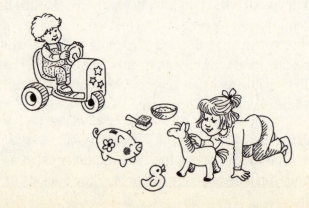

Uppity-Do Hairdressers

Take turns creating fun, goofy, or slick new dos at a pretend salon.

What You'll Need	All Ages	Babies	Toddlers	Preschoolers	School-Age Children
Pillow	🖑				
Hats	🖑				
Spray bottle with water	🖑				
Baby brush		🖑			
Hand mirror	🖑				
Wide-tooth comb			🖑	🖑	🖑
Hair accessories, such as ribbons, clips, elastic ponytail holders			🖑	🖑	🖑
Hair gel					🖑

Children can take turns styling one another's hair. Depending on the height of the stylist, have the customer sit on a pillow (for comfort), on a chair, or on the floor so the stylist can easily reach the hair. Put the styling supplies on a nearby table.

Babies

Because a baby's scalp and skull are fragile, it's best not to let your other children style a baby's hair. Instead, they can place a large hat on her head and gently take it off for a fun peekaboo game. Or you can be the stylist—babies don't need a full head of hair to be great customers! Mist their head with water and use a baby brush to gently brush their scalp or hair. Hold a mirror in front of their face so they can admire your handiwork.

Toddlers

Toddlers can hold a hand mirror and watch their playmates style their hair. They may especially enjoy accessories like hats or clips. When it's a toddler's turn to be the stylist, let him use a wide-tooth comb. Remind him to be gentle! Combing hair is a good exercise for his hand muscles.

Preschoolers

Let preschoolers use a spray bottle to wet their customer's hair. Then let them comb it out and add accessories to it.

School-Age Children

School-age children may want to try some advanced styling techniques on their customer's hair. Show them how to braid the hair or pull it into a ponytail. They may also choose to use hair gel to sculpt spikes or waves.

Checkup at the Doctor's Office

Kids will love being doctors and fixing boo-boos!

What You'll Need	All Ages	Babies	Toddlers	Preschoolers	School-Age Children
Books, magazines, and toys	🖐				
Blanket and pillow	🖐				
Doctor's kit items, such as Band-Aids, tongue depressors (Popsicle sticks), thermometer (straw), stethoscope (headphones), prescription pad (notepad), stickers, and scale			🖐	🖐	🖐
White adult-size T-shirt	🖐				
Large sheet of paper				🖐	
Crayons				🖐	
Tape				🖐	

Set up the play area to look like a doctor's office. Create a waiting room by setting out chairs, books, magazines, and toys. Make an examination room in part of the area by setting out a couple of chairs with a blanket and pillow on the floor. Gather items for a doctor's kit, then let kids take turns playing doctor and patient. Have the doctor wear a large, white T-shirt, then pretend to check the patient's temperature, listen to her heart, test her vision, put a Band-Aid on a cut, and even write a prescription!

Babies
Babies make great patients. Have the doctors count the baby's toes, look into her eyes, and make her smile. She will love the interaction and will begin to bond with her playmates.

Toddlers
When a toddler is the doctor, make requests such as, "Will you please check my ears? Where are my ears? How many ears do I have?" This is a fun way to teach toddlers about anatomy. To keep a toddler's attention while he is the patient, keep the "exam" action packed! For example, the doctor can ask him to crouch down to touch his toes and then jump up as high as he can.

Preschoolers
Preschoolers can design a vision test for their patients. Have them write a few letters on a large sheet of paper. Tape the paper to a wall, then the patients can take turns reading the letters out loud. For a more realistic vision test, the patient can block one eye with a hand while identifying the letters.

School-Age Children
School-age children can have fun writing prescriptions for the patients' pretend ills. For example, they can write, "Eat two cookies," and then sign the prescription with a flourish.

Host Tip
Make up a funny doctor's name for each child, like "Dr. It-Won't-Hurt-A-Bit" or "Dr. No-Shots."

Animal Hospital

Give some beloved plush animals a dose of TLC at this friend-operated animal hospital.

What You'll Need	All Ages	Babies	Toddlers	Preschoolers	School-Age Children
Plush animals	🖐				
Blanket	🖐				
Vet kit items, such as a stethoscope (headphones), otoscope (spoon), brush, and Band-Aids				🖐	🖐
Stickers			🖐		
Shoebox				🖐	🖐

While children round up some plush animals, set up some chairs in an area to be the waiting room. To create the examination room, lay a small blanket on the floor and place the vet kit nearby. Older children can take turns playing the veterinarian and the pet owner while younger children play the animal hospital staff.

Babies

Babies can be the waiting-room attendants. Let them sit on the floor among the plush animals. They may enjoy reaching for them, touching their soft fur, and gazing at their faces. Hold one close to a baby and make the animal's sounds. She'll enjoy listening to the noises.

Toddlers

Toddlers may enjoy being the vet assistant in charge of bringing the patients in and out of the examination room. Show them how to wrap each animal in a blanket. They can even place stickers on the animals to reward them for being brave during the examination!

Preschoolers and School-Age Children

Preschoolers and school-age children can take turns being the veterinarian and the pet owner. The vet can ask, "What happened to your pet? Has he eaten lately?" and then examine the animal using the vet kit. The vet can provide a diagnosis such as, "He needs a Band-Aid and rest!" The pet owners can ask questions such as, "How can I help my pet feel better?" Let them bring their pets home using a carrier fashioned from an open shoebox.

Planes, Trains, and Automobiles

With some imagination, children can really go places!

What You'll Need	All Ages	Babies	Toddlers	Preschoolers	School-Age Children
Large towels	🖐				
Couch cushions or pillows	🖐				
Fan	🖐				
Tissues			🖐		
Old keys				🖐	
Plastic plate					🖐

Here you'll find four transportation games you can play as a group, even though they are each geared toward specific age groups. After setting up each game, let children use their imaginations to create the experience: Where are they going? What do they see? What happens during the ride?

Babies

Babies will love playing "Train." Roll up two large towels per child lengthwise and lay them on the floor parallel to each other and about two feet apart. Have older children sit between the towels. Encourage them to bounce up and down as they make train noises like, *"Chugga, chugga, choo, choo!"* A baby can either sit in your arms or sit propped against rolled-up towels. Or he can get some tummy time by lying over a rolled-up towel.

Toddlers

Toddlers will enjoy "Plane." Place soft pillows or cushions in a line, one behind another, and have children sit on them. To feel as though you're soaring through the clouds, turn on a small fan in front of the first pillow. (Be sure the fan is out of reach of small hands.) Then encourage kids to hold out their arms like wings. A toddler may enjoy being the pilot on the first cushion. She can release tissues into the breeze from the fan. To the passengers, the tissues will look like passing clouds!

Preschoolers

"Car" is geared toward preschoolers! Set out pillows in two rows. They'll become seats for your car. Have a preschooler sit in the driver's seat and encourage other kids to climb in, too.

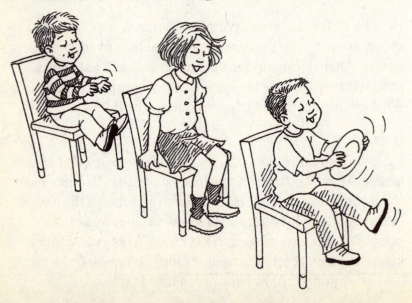

If you like, give a preschooler real car keys to start the "car." Have the driver act out putting on a seat belt, checking mirrors, beeping the horn, stopping at red lights, and so on.

School-Age Children

"Bus" is the perfect game for school-age children. Set out chairs or lay pillows on the floor to create rows of seats. Set a chair in front of the first row. Let a school-age child be the bus driver. Give her a plastic plate as a steering wheel, and have her open the bus door to let her friends on board. If she rides a bus to school, encourage her to teach her friends the rules of safe bus riding. If you like, sing "The Wheels on the Bus" with the other kids as your school-age child drives from stop to stop.

Walk on the Moon

Turn a living room into the surface of the moon and let kids explore!

What You'll Need	All Ages	Babies	Toddlers	Preschoolers	School-Age Children
Child-safe scissors	🖐				
Paper bags	🖐				
Stickers and crayons			🖐	🖐	🖐
String			🖐	🖐	🖐
Large and small sponges			🖐	🖐	🖐
Blankets and pillows	🖐				

Before you launch your astronauts into outer space, equip them properly: Create a space helmet for each child by cutting out a large square from the front of a paper bag. If the kids like, they can decorate their helmets as well as the baby's helmet with stickers and crayons, then they can place them over their heads. For moon shoes, use string to attach large sponges, like the kind used to wash a car, to the bottoms of preschoolers' and school-age children's feet. Use kitchen sponges for toddlers.

To create a rocket, set out four chairs to be the corners of a five-foot-by-five-foot square. Drape a blanket over the chairs. Invite children to lie on their backs inside the rocket, much as real astronauts are positioned during takeoff. Finally, create a moon surface while the kids wait to blast off by laying pillows and crumpled blankets on the floor as craters and rocks.

Babies

Lay the baby on her back on a blanket for a fun blastoff game. Give a countdown: "10, 9, 8, 7, 6, 5, 4, 3, 2, 1…" Then shout, "BLASTOFF!" and raise her to the sky. She'll love the anticipation and the motion!

Toddlers

When the rocket lands on the moon, encourage toddlers to navigate the surface. Walking in moon shoes around the craters and rocks will take concentration and will be good exercise for them!

Preschoolers and School-Age Children

What adventures will preschoolers and school-age children have on the moon? Encourage them to go on moonwalks, collect samples from the surface, take images of the moonscape, and repair space equipment. While playing, tell them the names of the planets of our solar system (Mercury, Venus, Earth, Mars, Jupiter, Saturn, Uranus, Neptune) and discuss what else astronauts do in space.

Host Tip
When making the rocket, use a crocheted blanket, if possible. The holes will give the appearance of stars.

Did You Know?
Moon Day is celebrated annually on July 20. It was on that day in 1969 that the first manned mission landed on the moon.

If the Shoe Fits

Kids will love trying on different styles and sizes of shoes in their own shoe store.

What You'll Need	All Ages	Babies	Toddlers	Preschoolers	School-Age Children
Various shoes	✋				
Shoeboxes				✋	
Tape measure or ruler					✋

Have children gather as many pairs of shoes as they like. Help them arrange the pairs in a designated area that will become their shoe store. Let them have fun trying on different pairs of shoes in different sizes.

Babies

Pick out shoes with textured soles, like a smooth dress shoe, a rubbery sneaker, and a rough work boot. Gently rub each sole on a baby's foot to stimulate the thousands of nerve endings there. She'll love the different sensations!

Toddlers

Toddlers are still mastering walking. If the toddler can walk skillfully, have him try on a few pairs of shoes to test his balance. He may want to slip on a pair of your shoes or an older friend's. For some pretend play, call him by the shoe owner's name. You can also pretend to be a customer sending him on a search for a specific pair of shoes, like blue shoes or shiny ones.

Preschoolers

Let preschoolers organize the shoe store by matching up the pairs of shoes and displaying them in any order they want. Perhaps they'll arrange the pairs by size or by color. They may also enjoy using shoeboxes to package sales. If preschoolers have trouble knowing which shoe goes on which foot, this activity is a great learning opportunity. Point out how one side of every shoe curves inward. Then encourage them to place a pair of shoes together, facing forward with the curves touching, in front of their feet. The left shoe will be in front of the left foot, and the right shoe will be in front of the right foot!

School-Age Children

Let school-age children measure everyone's feet with a tape measure or ruler. They can lay the tool on the floor and ask each person to stand next to it while they record the length. Who has the smallest feet? The largest? If they add the measurements together, what number do they get?

Host Tip

This activity may be a great time to teach preschoolers how to tie shoelaces. Here's a story to help your child remember the steps: "Two bananas were hanging from a vine. One day a silly monkey came by and crossed them over like an *X*. Then he jumped down, put one banana through the bottom half of the *X*, and pulled. Next, he made each banana into a loop and made another *X* with them. He put one banana loop under the *X* and pulled again. The little monkey was quite proud of his work and jumped and played the rest of the day."

Cool School Days

Let the learning begin in a pretend school!

What You'll Need	All Ages	Babies	Toddlers	Preschoolers	School-Age Children
Coloring books, paper, crayons, and books	🖐				
Chalkboard (or black construction paper and tape)				🖐	
Book bag			🖐		
Chalk				🖐	
Ruler				🖐	

Create a space to serve as a classroom. Set up a few work stations that include coloring books, paper, crayons, and books. You can even set up a small chalkboard, if you have one. (Or you can create a "chalkboard" by taping black construction paper to the wall.) Children will have fun teaching one another art, reading, and writing!

Babies

Babies may make the perfect students: They are both observant and curious. The "teachers" can entice babies' senses by sharing colorful pages from a book or by singing songs.

Toddlers

When it's a toddler's turn to be the teacher, help her get into character by giving her a bag to carry some books. She may want to hand out paper and crayons to her students. What does she want them to draw? Encourage her to call out ideas like "bird" or "tree."

Preschoolers

A great way for preschoolers to practice writing and identifying letters is for them to teach them to their playmates. Have a preschooler write his name on the chalkboard. Give him a ruler to point to each letter as he recites them to his students. Take this time to teach him how to spell simple words like *cat* and *dog*, then let him point out each letter to the students.

School-Age Children

School-age children can take attendance when they are the teacher. Have them call out each child's name. The students can respond, "Here!" To practice reading out loud, they can read a story to the students. Encourage the teacher to ask the students about the book. Who was in it? How did it end? Were there any silly parts in the story?

> When I was a child, my favorite thing to play was school. I used to prop up my baby sister on pillows and surround her with books and other students (my plush animals). I would read to her and show her pictures!
>
> —Lisa

Dining Out

Let children open their own restaurant complete with play
food and a menu.

What You'll Need	All Ages	Babies	Toddlers	Preschoolers	School-Age Children
Magazines			🖐	🖐	🖐
Child-safe scissors				🖐	🖐
Construction paper			🖐	🖐	🖐
Crayons			🖐	🖐	🖐
Glue sticks			🖐	🖐	🖐
Paper plates and napkins			🖐	🖐	🖐
Place mats			🖐	🖐	🖐
Plastic play food		🖐	🖐		
Notepad and pencil				🖐	
Apron					🖐
Pots, pans, and cooking utensils					🖐

Designate a space to serve as the restaurant. Children can search
through magazines to find images of food to cut out for the
menu. To make the menu, help children fold a sheet of construction paper lengthwise and widthwise to make four sections.
School-age children can label the sections "Drinks," "Dinners,"
"Side Dishes," and "Desserts." Have children glue each food
image onto the appropriate section. Finally, encourage kids to set
the table with paper plates and napkins. If you like, use the place
mats from "Trace a Place Mat" (see page 286).

Babies

Babies can patronize the restaurant. Set the baby in a highchair or bouncy seat and let playmates show her the menu. With a small gurgle or movement, she can indicate her choice, or the server can surprise her! Have the server bring play food the baby can explore.

Toddlers

Toddlers can take turns being a server and a patron. Challenge them to balance play food on plates when serving customers. No worries if they spill! When they're restaurant patrons, toddlers will enjoy making their own decisions by pointing to items on the menu. Encourage toddlers to order an item from each section.

Preschoolers

Preschoolers will enjoy being patrons, but may prefer working on the restaurant floor. Let them take turns greeting and seating guests and taking orders by jotting marks on a notepad. They can also bus the tables. Maybe they'll get a tip!

School-Age Children

School-age children can staff the kitchen and serve as the restaurant chef. Let them wear aprons and use some pots and pans as they pretend to prepare scrumptious foods in a designated "kitchen" area. A small table can serve as a counter, sink, or stove. They may also enjoy leaving the cooking to someone else as they take turns as patrons.

Let's Go Grocery Shopping

Open your kitchen cabinets and let children set up a grocery store.

What You'll Need	All Ages	Babies	Toddlers	Preschoolers	School-Age Children
Canned and boxed food items	🖐				
Play money			🖐	🖐	🖐
Paper bags	🖐				
Post-it notes and pencil				🖐	
Poster board					🖐
Crayons or magazines, child-safe scissors, and glue					🖐

Encourage children to find canned and boxed food in your kitchen cupboards. Or, if you prefer, set out a selection of items on the counter for them to choose from. (Supervise closely so the children don't handle breakable or hazardous items and so tiny fingers don't get pinched in the cupboard doors.) They can use the food to set up a grocery store on the kitchen table or the floor. Your shoppers will have fun selecting items, paying for them with play money, then loading and unloading them into and out of paper bags.

Babies

For babies older than six months, give them a few small food boxes to handle and stack. You also can create a small tower of boxes for them to knock over. If a baby is younger than six months, place him in his stroller for a walk around the grocery store to see the brightly colored items and watch the other children bustle about. Also try crumpling a paper bag near him. He'll react to the interesting sound.

Toddlers

Toddlers enjoy arranging objects, so let them stock the shelves. Can they make a tower of soup cans? Can they sort the canned objects from the boxed ones? Sorting is an early mathematical skill.

Preschoolers

Preschoolers can be grocery store clerks. They can help locate food items, bag them, and then check out the customers. Provide them with some play money to use as change for customer transactions. Although they can't calculate exact change, they can imitate transactions they have witnessed at the real grocery store. Make sure they give each customer a receipt (a Post-it Note) with either scribbles or handwritten numbers.

School-Age Children

School-age children can create a poster highlighting grocery store specials, using drawings or glued-on magazine cutouts of food. Have them work on the poster in the store so when customers walk by, they can inform them about the specials. Have them describe the items in enticing ways, such as, "These green beans are fresh," or, "This box of cereal has a toy inside it."

Parent Tip
The grocery store activity is a simple way to teach children about charity and giving. While the children are "shopping," ask them each to pick out one or two items to place in a special bag that you have set aside. Tell them that you'll bring the bag to a local food shelf, where it can go to a family in need.

> My son and nephew used to spend hours unloading all the soup cans from my cabinet and arranging them on the table. They had just as much fun putting them all back!
> —Lisa

Chapter 3

Music & Movement

I remember watching my four-month-old son as he used all his strength to roll over for the first time. My husband and I waited eagerly, whispering encouraging words. He pushed, he struggled, and finally…success! He lifted up his head and gave a smile that seemed to say, "This is only the beginning!"

—Lisa

Sometimes it seems that kids' bodies have minds of their own, especially when they start hopping and bopping to music. In this chapter, we provide engaging activities and games that focus on physical movement or musical creations—oftentimes both! Whether kids are singing and dancing to their own music video, playing homemade instruments, or striking energizing yoga poses, they will have fun moving their bodies and appreciating music of all kinds.

Morning Stretches

Start the day with these energizing stretches!

What You'll Need	All Ages	Babies	Toddlers	Preschoolers	School-Age Children
Plush animals			✋	✋	✋

Have the playmates sit on the floor. Toddlers, preschoolers, and school-age children will enjoy doing the stretches suggested below, and babies will enjoy stretching with a little help.

Babies
Lay the baby on her back. Playfully and gently grasp one hand and the opposite foot and stretch them out. Repeat this action with the other hand and foot. You can also try loosening up the hip muscles: In the same position, hold each leg and gently move the legs in a bicycling motion around and around.

Toddlers, Preschoolers, and School-Age Children
Show playmates how to do the following stretches:
- **Hello, Sun Stretch:** Sitting with your legs straight out in front of you, raise your arms above your head, then slowly reach for your feet.
- **Out-of-Bed Bend:** Sitting with your legs spread out to the sides, raise your arms above your head, then slowly bend to each side toward a foot.

- **Tickle Circle:** Sit in a circle with your legs straight out so your feet touch everyone else's. Reach forward and tickle one another's feet!

- **The Go-Go:** Find a partner, then sit facing each other with your legs straight out and your feet touching. Grab your partner's hands, then take turns leaning back while gently pulling your partner forward. If one partner is taller than the other, he will have to bend his legs while leaning forward.

- **The Up and About:** Stand up and hold a plush animal over your head. Bring the animal down to your toes, then stand back up and hold it straight out in front of you. Twist from side to side.

It's a Jungle Out There

This energetic activity will have playmates crawling, hopping, and prancing like wild animals.

What You'll Need	All Ages	Babies	Toddlers	Preschoolers	School-Age Children
Hula-Hoops (or pillows)	✋				

Arrange a Hula-Hoop (or pillow) for each child on the floor, spacing them about two feet apart. As a group, choose a wild animal, then have the children pretend to be the animal and move like it around the Hula-Hoops. They may need to hop, slither on their bellies, or crawl on all fours. Explain to them that the Hula-Hoops are hiding places where they can go if there's danger. When you say, "I hear something! Hide!" they should move into the nearest Hula-Hoop, crouch low, and stay still until you say all is clear. Repeat the game with another animal.

Babies

Team up with any babies and hold them face-out as you move like the animal. They'll love the movement and watching the other "animals" in action. To help build their vocabulary, say, "We're pretending to be a *bear*."

Toddlers

Animals have many ways of getting around—so do toddlers. Toddlers may enjoy lying on the ground and slithering like a snake or getting on all fours and strutting like a lion. If they need direction, point out how older playmates use their bodies to move like animals. For example, you could point out how someone holds their hands on their hips and lifts one knee to look like a flamingo.

Preschoolers and School-Age Children

Encourage preschoolers and school-age children to act out the motions of animals without naming them. Can anyone in the group guess what they are? If not, they can give clues such as, "This animal has a very long neck." Once someone recognizes the animal, everyone can act out its movements.

Shake It

Playmates will get in the groove with these homemade make-
'em-and-shake-'em percussion instruments.

What You'll Need	All Ages	Babies	Toddlers	Preschoolers	School-Age Children
Empty containers with lids, such as plastic bottles, plastic tubs, shoeboxes, coffee cans, and so on	✋				
Rattling materials, such as dried beans, pebbles, uncooked rice, dry cereal, cotton balls, marbles, and coins	✋				
Masking tape	✋				
Spoons				✋	✋

Give playmates empty containers with lids, such as plastic bottles, plastic tubs, small shoeboxes, coffee cans, and so on. Have
them pour dried beans, pebbles, or other rattling materials
into them, then help them secure the lids with tape. Then let
them shake away, making their own rhythms or following the
beat of their favorite music! *Note:* Supervise closely because
the small rattling materials could pose a choking risk for
younger children.

Babies
Make instruments for babies with containers that will be easy
to grasp, such as plastic bottles. They'll love making noise on

their own. If they are not able to hold the instrument, gently shake it close to them and move it slowly around them. They may follow it with their eyes as well as their ears.

Toddlers

Have toddlers pick a container and rattling material, then fill their containers for them. They can help secure the lids on the containers, though, if you put pieces of tape on the edge of the table for them to peel off and stick. This simple task will challenge their budding motor skills, as will shaking the instruments when they're finished.

Preschoolers and School-Age Children

Let older children experiment by filling different containers with different rattling materials to hear the different sounds they make. Have them look around the house for big and small containers made from plastic, cardboard, and wood. Encourage them to fill the containers with uncooked rice, dry cereal, cotton balls, marbles, or coins. They can also try banging on their instruments with spoons instead of shaking them.

Host Tip

As a special craft, help children make a rainstick—a South American instrument traditionally made of hollow cactus wood and lava pebbles. When the stick is tipped, the pebbles cascade down spines inside the tube, creating a sound like a rainshower. Here are the easy-to-follow steps to make your own rainstick:

1. Tape a piece of aluminum foil over one end of a gift-wrap tube. If you don't have a gift-wrap tube, tape several paper-towel tubes together.
2. Cut a piece of aluminum foil about two times as long as your tube and about six inches wide.
3. Twist and roll the foil into a thin strip, then curl it like a spring. Slide the curled foil into the tube.
4. Fill the tube with half a cup of dried beans or uncooked rice.
5. Tape a piece of foil over the second end of the tube.
6. Tip the finished rainstick to hear the gentle sound of a rainshower.

Pick a Move

This activity combines chance with imagination in order to get the group moving!

What You'll Need	All Ages	Babies	Toddlers	Preschoolers	School-Age Children
Deck of playing cards	✋				
Watch or clock	✋				

Remove the face cards from a deck of playing cards. Have the playmates sit on the floor in a circle and place the remaining cards face-down in the center. Have the first player choose a movement—like hopping on one foot, running in place, skipping, doing jumping jacks, crawling, or twirling around—then have her pick a card. The number on the card indicates how many seconds the player must do the movement. For instance, a child who chooses to do jumping jacks and picks a nine card must do jumping jacks for nine seconds. Use a watch or clock to time the children, or teach them to time seconds by counting, "One Mississippi, two Mississippi…" and so on. When the first player is done, the next player thinks of a movement and picks a card.

Babies

Babies can do this activity, too. When it's baby's turn, have older playmates choose a movement and a card for him. Then help baby walk, crawl, roll, or jump for the appropriate number of seconds. Have older playmates count each second aloud as a way to make it even more exciting.

Toddlers

Suggest a movement you know the toddlers can do, or if they have something in mind, let them go for it! Let the toddler pick a card and then count to that number together. If she draws a three, announce, "[Toddler's name] is going to show us how she can roll. She will roll for three seconds. Are you ready, [toddler's name]?" Have her playmates count the seconds as she performs.

Preschoolers and School-Age Children

Encourage preschoolers and school-age children to demonstrate moves they learned at school or in a class. For example, they may choose to tap dance or pretend to ice-skate. To make it a bit more challenging, ask older children to do their movements with their eyes closed or in a circle.

My preschooler loved when he picked a ten. Doing the movement for ten seconds while his siblings cheered him on was really fun for him!

—Lisa

Give Me an *A!*

Bring letters to life with this body-twisting activity.

What You'll Need	All Ages	Babies	Toddlers	Preschoolers	School-Age Children
Poster board	🖐				
Marker	🖐				
Blanket		🖐			

Before doing this activity, write the alphabet in capital letters on a sheet of poster board. Tell the children they can use it as a visual cue to help them shape their bodies into letters.

Babies

Lay the baby on a blanket and closely supervise as her older playmates work to form a letter with her body. For instance, they can raise the baby's arms wide above her head and hold her legs together to make a *Y*. Or they can team up with her to make a letter, such as if the baby and a playmate lie at angles and touch toes to create a *V*. If a baby is too young or just restless during the letter-building attempts, sit her close to the chart and point to the letters as her playmates make each letter with their bodies.

Toddlers

Toddlers may be starting to visually recognize letters. This activity will re-emphasize the shapes of the letters they know. Point to letters with simple, continuous lines, like *I* or *C*. Help them create these lines by standing them up straight like the *I* or helping them move their bodies and arms into the curve of the *C*.

Preschoolers and School-Age Children

Preschoolers and school-age children can look at the chart and choose which letters to form individually, as a pair, or with the help of the group. Can they come up with a formation for every letter? Let them use their imagination and team skills to tackle the challenge.

Host Tip
Take pictures of the kids as they form letters. What will they spell out?

Pop! Go Our Bodies

Gather around in a circle for a fun game that will have children popping and singing.

What You'll Need	All Ages	Babies	Toddlers	Preschoolers	School-Age Children
Bodies and voices	✋				

Hold hands and walk in a circle as you sing these lyrics to the tune of "Pop! Goes the Weasel." For each round, choose two children to name.

> *All around [child's name's] house,*
>   *[playmate's name] is watching.*
> *(S)he shouts, "Boo!"* (The child named in the first line shouts, "Boo!")
> *We count to two.* (Everyone counts to two and crouches close to the ground.)
> *Pop! Go our bodies!* (Release hands and everyone pops up, twirls, then drops down.)

Babies

For babies younger than eight months old, hold them as you walk. Support older babies under their arms and help them walk around in a circle. The activity will be great walking practice, and the song will reinforce babies' knowledge of playmates' names. Babies will love to hear their own names, too.

Toddlers, Preschoolers, and School-Age Children

Encourage toddlers, preschoolers, and school-age children to make special moves when it's time to pop. Let them create their own moves at first, but then teach them these fun jumping motions:

- **The Straight Jump:** Keep your body and legs as straight as possible as you jump in the air and land again.
- **The Tuck Jump:** Touch your hands to your knees while jumping.
- **The Straddle Jump:** Jump up and spread your legs apart.

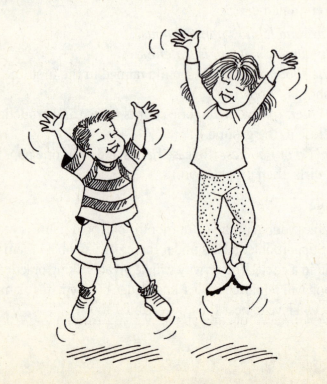

We've Got the Beat

What You'll Need	All Ages	Babies	Toddlers	Preschoolers	School-Age Children
Spoon and pot	🖐				
Rattle toys		🖐			

Have each child take a turn creating a beat with their hands, feet, or a spoon and pot while everyone else dances and moves to it. Tell them to freeze when the beat stops and move faster when the beat does.

Babies

Babies are learning to locate the source of noises. They may turn their heads to track the sound of the beat. They may also move their arms and bounce to the rhythm with or without help. Babies six months or older may enjoy making noise by shaking rattle toys. Help them shake a toy to a beat playmates can move to.

Toddlers

Reinforce how a toddler's body should move to the beat by saying, "The beat is very, very slow. Move your body slowly." Or "This beat is fast. Shake your body to the beat. Shake it fast!" Put your hands gently on his shoulders if he needs help remembering to freeze whenever the beat stops! When toddlers make the beat for their playmates, prompt them to slow down, speed up, and stop at various times.

Preschoolers and School-Age Children

Encourage preschoolers and school-age children to get creative with their movements. When the beat is a loud, slow banging, they may want to dance like giants. When the beat has quick, soft sounds, they may want to crawl like ants. Connecting sounds to animals or objects will boost their imaginations. When it is their turn to create the beat, perhaps they will do it to the beat of a familiar song or nursery rhyme.

> I play this game with my older children in the morning when I'm trying to get their shoes and coats on. They put their things on to my beat. If the beat is slow, they move slowly when zipping their coat up. When my beat is fast, they race to get their shoes on.
>
> —Lisa

Act It Out

Encourage children to act out simple nursery rhymes and children's songs.

What You'll Need	All Ages	Babies	Toddlers	Preschoolers	School-Age Children
Nursery rhyme books or CDs	✋				

Using books or CDs that feature nursery rhymes, help children find rhymes that inspire movement, such as "Jack Be Nimble" or "Jack and Jill." As you recite the rhymes out loud together (or play the CD), encourage the kids to add the coordinating actions.

Babies

Have fun moving with the babies by lifting them up and lowering them for "The Itsy-Bitsy Spider" and playfully lowering them to one side for "I'm a Little Teapot."

Toddlers

Toddlers may follow the motions you make with a baby or those older playmates make. Be sure to pick a few familiar rhymes they know, and perhaps say them slowly line by line so they have time to make each action.

Preschoolers and School-Age Children

Have preschoolers and school-age children partner up whenever possible, like in "Row, Row, Row Your Boat." They can face one another and hold hands as they lean forward and backward as in a rowing motion. You may also want them to leaf through the nursery rhyme book and pick one or two new ones to act out together, complete with movements to depict what is happening in the rhyme.

> **Did You Know?**
> The origins of most nursery rhymes reflect events in history. "Jack Be Nimble" is thought to be associated with the old tradition of candle leaping, which used to be featured at English fairs.

Soaring with Scarves

Use silk scarves to get kids' minds and bodies moving.

What You'll Need	All Ages	Babies	Toddlers	Preschoolers	School-Age Children
Silk (or cotton) scarves (available at your local craft store)	🖐				
Music	🖐				

Give each child a scarf, turn on some music, and let the children use their imaginations to move their bodies and their scarves however they want. Change the song every thirty seconds and have them slow down or speed up their movements, depending on how the song makes them feel.

Babies
Babies older than six months may enjoy holding the scarf in their hands and waving it. If they are younger, hold the scarf near their face and gently move it to the beat of the music.

Toddlers
Encourage toddlers to try new movements with their scarf, such as holding it low to the ground or high to the sky. You can also have them twirl with their scarves, or show them how to scrunch the scarf into a ball and throw it into the air. Can they catch it as it drifts back to the ground?

Preschoolers

Preschoolers probably won't need any instruction as they skip or gallop with the scarf to fast music. During a slower song, though, have them try this relaxing technique: Have them hold the scarf in front of their face, take a deep breath in, and then exhale to blow the scarf up.

School-Age Children

While dancing, school-age children can have fun swirling their scarves in front of them in the shape of a circle. Can they form the letters of their names? For example, can they move the scarf quickly down and to the right to make an *L*?

Yoga

Yoga is a great way to help kids of all ages to focus and relax.

What You'll Need	All Ages	Babies	Toddlers	Preschoolers	School-Age Children
Bath towels	✋				

In a room with a lot of open space, show children how to do the yoga poses on page 97. Because the Cobra and Child's Poses require lying on the floor, it's best to do this activity in a carpeted room. If the floor isn't carpeted, have the children do these poses on a bath towel. Below you'll find some age-appropriate ways children can enjoy these yoga poses.

Babies

Even a young baby can enjoy yoga! If the baby can lift his head, lay him on his belly and watch him move into a version of the Cobra pose as he raises his head and shoulders. (If he's not yet able to lift his head, his body will still benefit from the tummy time.) While older playmates practice the Down Dog pose, the baby will enjoy looking up at their upside-down faces as he sits or lies on his back nearby.

Toddlers

Toddlers may have little trouble moving into the Cobra and Down Dog poses. The Cobra pose builds on skills they learned as babies (raising their heads and upper bodies while on their bellies). The Down Dog pose builds on a position a toddler may have used while learning to stand from a crawling position or when seated on the floor. The Child's Pose may take a bit of practice, though. There are several steps that require careful listening. You can help by telling the toddlers to kneel down and then sit on their heels. Hold the toddler's feet in this position while she tries to lean forward and put her chest and head on the floor.

Preschoolers and School-Age Children

Preschoolers and school-age children have the strength and focus to control their movements. Encourage them to hold each pose as they slowly count to ten. This will let them fully reap the pose's cognitive and physical benefits.

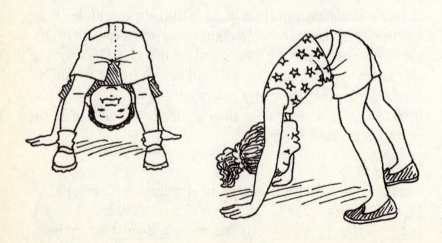

Yoga Poses

Cobra
Cognitive Benefit: Creates a feeling of strength.

Physical Benefit: Strengthens the back and the whole upper body.

How to Do It: Lie on your belly with your legs together and your face parallel to the floor. Bend your elbows so your forearms are on the floor and tucked next to your body. Push down on your forearms and slowly raise your head and chest.

Down Dog
Cognitive Benefit: Helps you stay focused.

Physical Benefit: Sends blood to the head for a burst of energy.

How to Do It: Stand with your feet hip-width apart. Bend at the waist and place your hands on the floor, keeping your back straight. Gaze behind you between your legs. (This pose has been modified for children.)

Child's Pose
Cognitive Benefit: Creates a feeling of safety.

Physical Benefit: Relaxes entire body.

How to Do It: Kneel on the floor with your legs and feet together, then sit back on your heels. Keeping your back straight, bend at the waist to place your forehead on the floor and stretch your arms straight out in front of you.

Aquapella

Drip, drop, plish, plosh, burble, babble—kids can create "music" with water!

What You'll Need	All Ages	Babies	Toddlers	Preschoolers	School-Age Children
Towels	✋				
Baking pan		✋			
Plastic cup			✋		
Drinking straw			✋		
Drinking glasses				✋	
Metal spoon				✋	
Plastic bottles					✋

Tell children they're going to make "music" with water, and they'll each play a different "instrument." Do this activity in your kitchen, where you can find all the materials and you won't have to worry about making a mess. (You still might want to keep some towels handy, though.)

Babies

If the baby is six months or older, pour about an inch of water in a baking pan and place it on the highchair tray. Encourage the baby to slap the water. It won't be long until she's splashing and creating her own unique percussion sound. If the baby is younger than six months, guide her hands to help her slap the water.

Toddlers

Fill a plastic cup halfway with water and give toddlers straws.
Show them how to blow into the water with the straw to create
bubbles and a silly sound. (You may need to remind them that
while it's fun to do this "musical technique" now, it's not something they should do every time they drink from a straw!)

Preschoolers

Help preschoolers fill three glasses with water: one glass
almost to the top, the second halfway, and the third with only
a bit. Place the glasses on a table. Preschoolers can gently tap
the side of each glass with a metal spoon. Note how the sound
changes in each glass, depending on how much water it holds.
Which one makes the highest sound? Maybe they'll be able to
play simple tune like "Mary Had a Little Lamb" while they tap
the glasses.

School-Age Children

Have school-age children fill three plastic bottles with varying
levels of water. Show them how to make music by perching
their lips on the edge of the bottle opening and blowing gently.
Have them blow into all three and note how the sound changes.
If you have different-size bottles, have the children experiment
with their sound, too.

New Musical Chairs

We've taken the competitiveness out of this traditional game and added more fun.

What You'll Need	All Ages	Babies	Toddlers	Preschoolers	School-Age Children
Chairs (one for each child)	✋				
Tape	✋				
Photos (one of each child)	✋				

Set up the chairs back to back in an open area. Tape a photo of each child to each chair. Sing a song of your choice to start everyone walking or dancing around the chairs. When you yell, "Stop!" each child must hurry to sit on the chair with his or her respective photo. After a few rounds, change the order of the chairs or the photos.

Babies

Sway and move to the beat of the song as you march around with the baby in your arms. Feeling your movement and hearing you sing is a great way for a baby to experience the joy of music. When you say, "Stop!" the baby will enjoy the hustle and bustle of everyone scrambling for their chairs.

Toddlers

Encourage toddlers to make silly movements as they go around the chairs. Can they jump, tiptoe, or trot? Can they move slowly or quickly to match the beat of the song? When it's time to find their chair, they may end up waiting to see which chair is empty after older playmates have found their places. To help them understand that the photos designate each child's chair, point to his photo and say, "Who is that? Whose chair is this?"

Preschoolers and School-Age Children

Challenge older children to think of other fun rules for this new version of musical chairs. Perhaps they'll suggest you arrange the chairs farther apart, or perhaps they'll tape the photos facedown so players must lift them one by one to find their chairs.

Pop Stars

Have aspiring pop stars over to play? They can perform in their own music videos!

What You'll Need	All Ages	Babies	Toddlers	Preschoolers	School-Age Children
Favorite music	🖑				
Dress-up clothes, such as hats and scarves	🖑				
"Microphones," such as spoons, toothbrushes, hairbrushes, and so on			🖑	🖑	🖑
Camcorder or other recording device	🖑				

Play children's favorite music or ask them to sing a song for you. Give them pretend microphones, and encourage them to dress up using hats, scarves, or other fun clothes. Each child can take a turn singing, humming, or cooing into a microphone like a pop star performing in a music video or concert. If possible, capture the performance with a camcorder or other recording device, then watch or listen to it as a group.

Babies

No doubt, the sound of voices is one of a baby's favorite things, so he'll love to listen to everyone sing. But make sure he gets in on the action, too. If he tries to gurgle or make sounds, mimic them back to him. He'll enjoy this interaction. During the performance, he can be center stage while one of his playmates helps him dance.

Toddlers

Toddlers may be happy simply blowing into the microphone, or they may be ready to sing a few notes of their favorite song. Remind the toddler of the lyrics by singing a few words then pausing to let her guess what comes next. See if she will finish the lyrics after a few tries!

Preschoolers and School-Age Children

Let older children take the lead with the performance. Encourage them to choose a song and help their playmates learn the words. They may even want to make up a dance routine or body movements to go along with the song.

> My children love to perform. My job is to introduce them. I make a big deal out of it, saying, "And now, ladies and gentlemen, I would like to introduce the amazingly talented Kyle and the sensational Brooke!" They get a kick out of it and perform their little hearts out!
>
> —Heather

Little Gymnasts

Get kids moving with balancing, jumping, and tumbling exercises!

What You'll Need	All Ages	Babies	Toddlers	Preschoolers	School-Age Children
Exercise mats (or a mattress)	✋				
Bath towel		✋			
Masking tape			✋		

Below you'll find some age-appropriate gymnastics for children. Be sure to supervise closely and use exercise mats (or a mattress) for safety.

Babies

Here's a fun "floor exercise" for babies at least three months old: Lay them on their back on a mat or bath towel and encourage them to reach for their toes. Put brightly colored socks on their feet and slowly raise their feet up so they are in view. Can the babies reach for them?

Toddlers

Help toddlers do a logroll: Have them lie horizontally across the mat with their arms straight over their heads so they look like logs. Encourage them to roll to the end of the mat in this position. Also, place a few X marks with masking tape about one foot apart on the floor. Suggest that the children try to jump from one to another.

Preschoolers

Help preschoolers do a forward somersault on the mat. Show them how to squat with their hands on the mat in front of them. Have the preschooler tuck his head as if he's looking at his belly-button, then tell him to use his legs to push up into a roll.

School-Age Children

Teach school-age children how to do a handstand. Slide the mat close to a wall. Have them face the wall and place their hands palms down on the mat. Help them kick their legs up against the wall. Proper position requires that knees and arms are locked, toes are pointed, and neck is tucked. Be sure to supervise closely.

Dancing with Feeling

Let children express themselves with some creative dance moves!

What You'll Need	All Ages	Babies	Toddlers	Preschoolers	School-Age Children
Variety of music	✋				

In a large, open space, play a variety of music, like big band, classical, pop, country, and lullabies. While the music plays, call out different feelings, such as "Happy!" or "Sad!" and encourage children to express each of those feelings through dance. If they need direction, here are some examples:

- **Sad:** Slump your shoulders and make a sad face.
- **Happy:** Throw your arms in the air and grin.
- **Sneaky:** Tiptoe or creep slowly.
- **Frustrated:** Stomp your feet and yell.
- **Silly:** Spin in circles and make funny faces.
- **Excited:** Make quick twists and turns.
- **Sleepy:** Make slow, drawn-out movements.

Babies

Baby will enjoy the movement and music as you dance while holding him. Babies love to study faces, so be sure to make exaggerated expressions for each feeling. He may try to mimic you!

Toddlers

Expressing themselves through dance will reinforce the different emotions toddlers are beginning to identify. To get them started, ask, "What does it feel like to be happy? Do you feel like jumping up and down?" or, "What do you feel like doing when you're sleepy? Do you rub your eyes?" Demonstrate the movements and encourage them to join in. They may also watch older playmates and mirror their movements.

Preschoolers

Preschoolers may discover that dance is a good way to communicate feelings they have trouble expressing in words. For example, they may find it difficult to express anger or sadness. Encourage them to come up with different dance moves to express those feelings in appropriate ways.

School-Age Children

Have school-age children call out a few feelings for everyone to dance to. Challenge them to listen to the music and identify a feeling that matches its tone and mood. Does a country ballad sound sad? Does a big band tune feel cheerful?

Bounce to the Beat

This activity will challenge kids' balance as they bounce to the beat!

What You'll Need	All Ages	Babies	Toddlers	Preschoolers	School-Age Children
Medium-size balls (about 12 inches in diameter)			🖐	🖐	🖐
Exercise ball		🖐			
Music	🖐				

In a large, open space, have toddlers, preschoolers, and school-age children each sit on a ball. Play a variety of music with different tempos, and challenge playmates to keep their balance as they bounce to the beats.

Babies

Hold the baby while you sit on an exercise ball. (If you don't have a ball, hold the baby on your lap as you sit on a chair.) If she is younger than four months, face her toward you and hold her so her head is over your shoulder. If she is older and has more neck control, hold her face out so she can see her playmates. Bounce to the beat of the music. The action will stimulate a calming reflex that may put her right to sleep!

Toddlers

Keeping balance on the ball will be a new challenge for toddlers. To help them practice balancing, have them sit on their ball near a wall they can use as support. If they need more assistance, hold them under their arms as they sit on the ball, and raise and lower their bodies to create the bouncing effect. Make sure to bounce fast during an upbeat tempo and slowly for a gentle rhythm.

Preschoolers and School-Age Children

For an additional challenge, see if preschoolers and school-age children can clap their hands or slap their knees while bouncing. It will be harder than they think! Because they are growing tall, their legs will have to bend closely to their torsos in order to stay on the ball.

Invisible Baseball

You won't need any equipment for this fun movement game!

What You'll Need	All Ages	Babies	Toddlers	Preschoolers	School-Age Children
Imaginations!	✋				

In an open space, tell the playmates it's baseball time, but you're going to play with invisible equipment! Everyone—even a baby—can participate. Take some time to teach older children the playing techniques below, but you may need to help younger children make the motions. For each turn, assign a pitcher, batter, and fielders, depending on the number of players. Encourage the children to play, and cheer on their pretend plays!

Pitching
Have the pitcher pretend she's holding a baseball in her hands. Her fingers and thumbs should be stretched out and curved around the ball. Teach her to make an overhand throw by pulling her throwing arm back with elbow bent, then springing it forward as she releases the ball.

Batting

It takes a lot of practice to hold a bat, let alone swing it, so this a great way to get ready for real baseball. Have the batter pretend to hold a bat by lining up his knuckles on the handle with his dominant hand on top. He can stand sideways on home plate with his head facing forward, hold the bat behind his shoulders, and swing out in front of him as the pitch approaches. After a hit, the batter can run the bases. (You can set up some checkpoints for the bases, or you can simply let him run in a circle.)

Fielding

Encourage the fielder to watch the batter closely to know when a hit is coming her way. Have her pretend to wear a mitt on her nondominant hand, stretching her fingers wide to open the mitt and closing the thumb to the fingers to catch the ball. Using her dominant hand, she can retrieve the ball from the mitt, then throw it to a base to stop the runner or throw it back to the pitcher.

Walk in My Steps

With this activity, kids will understand what it means to walk in someone else's footsteps!

What You'll Need	All Ages	Babies	Toddlers	Preschoolers	School-Age Children
Felt (2 sheets per child)	✋				
Chalk	✋				
Music	✋				

To begin, have each playmate stand on a sheet of felt while you or an older child traces the footprints with chalk. (Hold babies under their arms if they are not old enough to stand on their own.) Repeat on another sheet of felt so each child makes two sets of footprints. Encourage playmates to place their feet in different positions for each tracing. They can point their feet outward or inward, stand with feet together or spread apart, position one foot above the other, or even stand on one foot. When you're done tracing, choose an open space on the floor and lay all the felt sheets in a long path. Turn on some lively music and have the kids move from one set of footprints to the next, placing their feet in the proper positions.

Babies

For babies who aren't walking on their own yet, hold them under their arms or by the hands as they "walk" through the footprint path. They may not put their feet in the right positions, but they'll love taking their own steps. Otherwise, you can hold the baby in your arms as you walk and hop through the path, stepping to the music.

Toddlers

Toddlers may try to speed through the path, but encourage them to take their time and study the position of each different set of footprints so they can match it. Say, "See how this foot points out and this foot points in? Can you put your feet that way, too?"

Preschoolers

Add some arm movements to give preschoolers an extra challenge as they walk through the prints. Can they hold their hands above their head and clap to the beat of the music while stepping into the prints? This may also be a good time to practice telling left from right by having preschoolers say, "Left!" or, "Right!" as they put each respective foot in a print.

School-Age Children

School-age children can arrange the felt pieces in a new path. They may want to shuffle the order of the footprints, make a circle or square with the pieces, or space them farther apart so playmates need to jump from one to the other and land as the footprints dictate.

Clap! Snap! Stomp!

This noisy activity is a great way to channel children's energy.

What You'll Need	All Ages	Babies	Toddlers	Preschoolers	School-Age Children
Bodies!	🖐				

Teach playmates the following chant and do the actions together:

> *Clap, clap, clap—my hands can do that part.*
> (Clap hands in rhythm.)
> *Snap, snap, snap—my fingers are so fast.*
> (Snap fingers in rhythm.)
> *Stomp, stomp, stomp—my feet can keep the beat.*
> (Stomp feet in rhythm.)
> *La, la, la—do you hear me now?*
> (Turn around in a circle.)

Next, call out one child's name and say, "Break it down!" That child gets to move and make sounds however she likes, then everyone else copies her. After a few seconds, say, "Freeze, please!" At that point, everyone must stand still and be quiet. Begin the chant again, choosing a different name next time for the "breakdown."

Babies

Babies will enjoy doing the actions with help. Hold your hands over your head and bring them together to show baby how to clap. If the baby is older than six months, he may love to clap by himself. Whether sitting or lying down, help the baby stomp by lifting his legs up and down. Don't forget to give the baby a turn to "break it down" and be the leader!

Toddlers

Chances are, toddlers may need help learning how to snap. Hold your hands in front of them and snap in slow motion, showing them how the middle finger touches the top of the thumb and then slides down. Help position their fingers for a snap. Even if they don't make much of a sound, encourage their efforts!

Preschoolers

Preschoolers will love this silly, noisy activity, so the challenge will be composing themselves when it's time to be still and quiet. If necessary, touch them on the shoulder when you give the command to freeze.

School-Age Children

When it's their turn to be the leader for the breakdown, have school-age children make sounds not with their voices, but with their bodies. They can slap their knees or rub the carpet with their feet. Encourage them to teach their playmates new movements to do.

Hokey-Pokey Friends

Everyone can "shake it all about" in this fun variation of a traditional tune!

What You'll Need	All Ages	Babies	Toddlers	Preschoolers	School-Age Children
A group of playmates!	✋				

Have children stand in a circle. If any babies are present who can stand with support, help them join the circle. Otherwise, hold a baby as you stand in the circle. Sing "The Hokey-Pokey" as a group, replacing each verse's body part with a child's name. For example, if one child's name is Emily, sing:

We put Emily in. (She runs into the middle of the circle.)
We put Emily out. (She runs back to her spot in the circle.)
We put Emily in. (She runs into the middle of the circle.)
And she shakes it all about. (She shakes her whole body.)
We do the hokey-pokey, and we turn ourselves around.
     (Everyone turns around in a circle.)
That's what it's all about! (Everyone claps to the beat of each word.)

Repeat the song, using each playmate's name. When it's the baby's turn, hold him as you move in and out of the circle, and gently sway from side to side when it's time to "shake." Make sure you take a turn, too. After everyone has had a turn, repeat the song once more, using "the whole group" as the subject!

Ring Those Bells

Playmates will enjoy making these bell wands, but they'll really love conducting their very own bell choir!

What You'll Need	All Ages	Babies	Toddlers	Preschoolers	School-Age Children
Paper-towel tubes	🖐				
Paint or crayons	🖐				
Clear contact paper		🖐			
Hole punch	🖐				
Various craft bells (2 per child)	🖐				
Yarn	🖐				

Give toddlers, preschoolers, and school-age children each a paper-towel tube to decorate with paint and crayons. Have them decorate tubes for any babies as well. Wrap the baby's decorated tube in clear contact paper in case she mouths it. Punch a small hole at both ends of each tube, then tie a bell to each hole with yarn. If you use different styles and sizes of bells, your bell choir will have a variety of tones. Once the bell wands are complete, each child can take a turn as the conductor. He can stand in front and point to a playmate when he wants her to ring her bells.

Babies

The bell wand is perfect for babies just learning to grasp objects. Let them shake it to hear the bells. When it's a baby's turn to be the conductor, sit her on your lap and move her arms to point to her playmates. After a few tries, see if she'll swing her arms on her own. Prompt the other children to play whenever they see her move. She'll love realizing that the kids ring the bells according to her movements!

Toddlers

Toddlers will enjoy standing in front of their playmates and pointing to the bells they want to hear. Depending on how fast they point, they can control the tempo of the choir. Encourage toddlers to move their arms fast when they want the bells to ring quickly and move their arms slowly when they want playmates to slow down.

Preschoolers

How can preschoolers make their bells ring besides shaking the wand? Can they tap the bells with their fingers or roll the wand back and forth on the ground? Have preschoolers pick a new technique, teach it to the choir, then lead them in a performance.

School-Age Children

Encourage school-age children to perform a solo of a simple tune such as "Jingle Bells" or "Mary Had a Little Lamb." As an extra challenge, have them conduct the choir to create a specific tune together. They may want to sing the song as they point to each playmate, helping them follow the tune.

Chapter 4

Outdoor Adventures

I happily take my kids outside every chance I get. Where else can they burn off energy, make a mess, and discover countless new things? We stomp in rain puddles, follow tracks in the snow, and study clouds for dinosaurs and cars.

—Lisa

There's a world of fun just outside your door. In this chapter, we include classic and new outdoor games that are fun for every age group. We also include a variety of special experiences kids can have only outdoors, such as searching for nature's treasures, studying the stars and clouds, and getting soaked with the sprinkler. The hard part may be getting the children to come back inside after a long day of playing and exploring!

Strollin' through Nature

Help children explore and collect natural treasures.

What You'll Need	All Ages	Babies	Toddlers	Preschoolers	School-Age Children
Paper bags			🖐	🖐	🖐
Glue stick				🖐	
Construction paper				🖐	
Markers				🖐	
Binoculars					🖐
Notebook and pencil					🖐

Give each child a paper bag, then take a walk through your neighborhood or a park. Have children use the bags to collect nature items, like flowers, rocks, and pinecones.

Babies

Nature provides a world of stimulation for babies. Talk to the babies about their surroundings. Point out a colorful flower, a smooth rock, or chirping birds. Encourage other children to describe what they see to the babies as well.

Toddlers

Toddlers will love picking up items and dropping them in their bags. Help build their vocabulary by identifying what they put in their bags. For example, say, "You found a green leaf. Can you say 'green leaf'?"

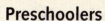

Preschoolers

Describe an object in the preschoolers' sight and have them guess what it is. For example, say, "I spy something green," to describe grass. Feel free to give them plenty of hints. They can take turns describing an object and having you or another child guess what it is. When you get home, help them glue the nature finds onto large sheets of construction paper. If you like, help them identify and label each object.

School-Age Children

School-age children can use binoculars to "collect" sightings of nature objects out of their normal sight, like a bird in a treetop or a butterfly on the far side of a field. If you like, give them notebooks to record what they observe on the walk.

Host Tip

To prepare for your nature walk, take a trip to your local library and check out nature guides on your area.

Ball In, Out, and About

This silly game will bring some music and action to your outdoor time.

What You'll Need	All Ages	Babies	Toddlers	Preschoolers	School-Age Children
Hula-Hoop (or two)	✋				
Foam balls	✋				
Marker			✋		

Lay a Hula-Hoop on the ground and have the kids sit around it. Give each child a foam ball of any size. Sing the following song to the tune of "The Hokey-Pokey" and follow the indicated movements:

> *You put the ball in the circle.*
>   (Hold the ball to the ground inside the Hula-Hoop.)
> *And you take the ball right out.*
>   (Hold the ball outside the Hula-Hoop.)
> *You put the ball in the circle.*
>   (Hold the ball inside the Hula-Hoop.)
> *And you shake it all about.* (Shake the ball as hard as you can.)
> *We do the bally-bally* (Stand up.)
> *And we give the ball a throw* (Throw the ball in the air.)
> *Hey, ball, where did you go?* (Chase the ball.)

Have the children run to collect their balls and gather back around the Hula-Hoop as quickly as they can.

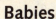

Babies

Babies will need partners for this activity. For babies six months or older, give them easy-to-grasp balls and guide them through the movements. They'll soon anticipate the actions and may try to release the ball on cue. Applaud their efforts! Hold younger babies while you perform the actions. They'll enjoy the movements and the song.

Toddlers

It won't take many rounds until the toddlers join in on the movements and belt out some of the song lyrics. Make their balls extra special: Use a marker to draw smiley faces on both sides. This way, toddlers can practice their tracking skills and find their balls quickly as they roll away.

Preschoolers and School-Age Children

To challenge preschoolers and school-age children, place another Hula-Hoop on the ground about five feet away from the first one. When it's time to toss their balls into the air, they can aim for the second Hula-Hoop. This exercise is a good precursor to skills required to play basketball and baseball. Preschoolers and school-age children can also try to catch their balls after they throw them in the air.

Sand Discoveries

Sand has a wonderful texture that most children love to feel running through their fingertips or squishing between their toes. Let children experiment with sand using different items.

What You'll Need	All Ages	Babies	Toddlers	Preschoolers	School-Age Children
Sandbox			✋	✋	✋
Sand toys, such as funnels, shovels, and pails			✋	✋	✋
Clear plastic bottle		✋			
Rocks or small sticks					✋

Set up a sandbox outside, then have the children use different objects to play with the sand. (If you don't have a sandbox, you can make one by adding sand—available at landscaping centers—to a large kiddie pool. Or you can use a sandbox at a local park.)

Babies

Babies love to discover new textures. For babies younger than six months, trickle a little sand from your hand over their hands. (Make sure none of the sand gets in their mouths.) For older babies, half-fill clear plastic bottles with sand; close them tightly; and let babies shake the bottles, roll them, and turn them upside down to watch the sand move.

Toddlers

Hold a funnel over a pail and show toddlers how to fill the funnels with sand by using shovels or cups. Toddlers will enjoy watching the sand drain into the pail. You also can give them a small amount of water to mix with the sand to see how the consistency changes.

Preschoolers

Show preschoolers how to make towers by filling pails with sand, packing the sand down, and quickly flipping the pails over on the ground. Challenge them to build sand castles by making towers next to each other.

School-Age Children

School-age children may enjoy setting up a sand town with roads, rivers, mountains, and bridges. They can use rocks to outline a road or small sticks to create a bridge. If they like, they can make a "drip castle": After they build a sand castle, show them how to make loose fists with one hand and then slowly pour a little wet sand through their fists and onto the sides of a sand castle. The water will make the sand "glob" together, creating a cool texture!

Host Tip

If you can't go outside, fill a shoebox with sand for each child and use measuring cups or small plastic cups as buckets. Make sure to lay a tarp or blanket to protect the floor!

> My son and his friend figured out how to create a sand volcano. They built a large mountain and buried a hose underneath the surface. When they turned on the water, the volcano erupted!
>
> —Heather

Welcome to Water World

This water-play activity is perfect for a warm day.

What You'll Need	All Ages	Babies	Toddlers	Preschoolers	School-Age Children
Bowls or buckets	✋				
Water "tools," such as sponges, ladles, funnels, spoons, paintbrushes, spray bottles, rocks, and measuring cups	✋				

Go outside and fill a small bowl or bucket with water for each child. Then let them explore what they can do with the water!

Babies

Position babies near bowls of water. For babies six months or older, dip ladles in the water and show them how to fill and empty them. For younger babies, let them see and hear water pouring into the bowls, feel water sprinkle on their hands, and taste drops of clean water in their mouths.

Toddlers

Toddlers' sense of discovery makes water play exciting. Let them experiment with colanders, funnels, or even plastic cups with several holes poked into the bottom. Show them how to fill in the objects with water and watch them drain out.

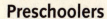

Preschoolers

It will be fun for preschoolers to discover that water can move in different ways. Fill small spray bottles. How far can the preschoolers get the stream of water to reach? Mark the distance with small rocks and have them try again. Later, fill large bowls with some water and give them each a paintbrush or large spoon to stir the water in a circular motion. How fast can they get the water to swirl? After they stop stirring, how long does the water continue to move?

School-Age Children

Sharpen school-age children's measuring and predicting skills. Have them predict the number of cups it'll take to fill their bowls, then see if they're right. Then have them predict the number of rocks they can add to their bowls of water before the water overflows. At the end of the activity, have the school-age children refill their bowls and set them someplace where they won't be disturbed. Ask them to predict how much water will be left in the bowls after a week has passed.

Stargazing

On a clear summer night, head outside to view the sky.

What You'll Need	All Ages	Babies	Toddlers	Preschoolers	School-Age Children
Large blanket	🖐				
Celestial map or book on constellations					🖐
Flashlight					🖐
Red tissue paper					🖐

Find a spot to stargaze, whether it be your own backyard or a public park. Avoid sitting directly under streetlights. The farther you are from city lights, the more you'll see. (If you can't find a starry-enough sky, modify this activity into a visit to a planetarium.) Spread a large blanket for your friends as you stargaze. There are approximately five thousand stars visible to the naked eye, and children will love to talk about those they see.

Babies

The stars may be too dim for babies to see, but they'll enjoy listening to the nature sounds. Lay the babies on their backs. Point to the stars and talk with them about all the nighttime noises they hear.

Toddlers

Toddlers will find an outdoor nighttime activity exciting! If the moon is out, ask them if they can point to the brightest object in the sky. Entice their imaginations by asking if they can see the "Man on the Moon" and what he may be doing up there. Hold their hands to point to the stars and count them together.

Preschoolers

Help preschoolers find a few popular stars and constellations, like the North Star (Polaris) and the Big Dipper (part of Ursa Major). Tell them the stories behind the constellation names (which may require some research beforehand). Encourage them to find their own constellations and create stories about them.

School-Age Children

School-age children will enjoy using a celestial map to identify a constellation. To help them see the stars in the book without obscuring their friends' view of the night sky, have them place red tissue paper over their flashlights.

> **Did You Know?**
> On the moon, it's three times as hot during the day and three times as cold at night as it is on Earth.

Hungry Wolf

How hungry is the wolf? Kids will be tempted to find out during this action-packed game.

What You'll Need	All Ages	Babies	Toddlers	Preschoolers	School-Age Children
Hungry wolves!	✋				

Each child will have a turn playing the wolf. The wolf should stand with his back to the others. The rest of the children will stand in a line facing the wolf about thirty feet away. Each child will take a turn asking the wolf, "Mr. Wolf, what time is it?" The wolf will respond with any time he chooses. If he says, "One o'clock," each child moves one step forward. If he says, "Nine o'clock," each child moves nine steps forward. He can also reply at any time with, "It's lunchtime!" At that point, the players must run back to their starting places before the wolf reaches them.

Babies

The babies will love to be in someone's arms during this game. Make sure to count the steps out loud as you move. Expect squeals and smiles as everyone rushes back when the wolf says it's lunchtime!

Toddlers

Watch toddlers as they begin to anticipate the moves of this game. They may jump with anticipation when they hear, "It's lunchtime!" When it's their turn to be the wolf, you can either prompt them to say a certain time or give them two times to choose from.

Preschoolers

Instead of taking steps, preschoolers can challenge themselves by hopping on one foot or jumping with both. Tell them to choose a mode that's fast enough to escape the hungry wolf!

School-Age Children

School-age children are able to associate the time of day with various activities. When it's their turn to play wolf, encourage them to provide a time and a corresponding action. For instance, they may respond, "It's eight o'clock, and time to get dressed." They could even act out the motions!

The Backyard Parade

March to your own beat as the kids create a friendly marching band!

What You'll Need	All Ages	Babies	Toddlers	Preschoolers	School-Age Children
Plastic bucket and stick			🖐	🖐	🖐
Plastic bottle with pebbles			🖐	🖐	🖐
Plastic plates			🖐	🖐	🖐
Paper-towel tubes			🖐	🖐	🖐
Spoons		🖐			
Old T-shirts				🖐	
Sticks				🖐	🖐

Help children make musical instruments from items found around the house. They can make a drum from a bucket and a stick; a maraca from a plastic bottle filled with pebbles; cymbals from two plastic plates; or a trumpet, flute, or clarinet from a paper-towel tube. Then the children can parade around the yard, playing their makeshift instruments.

Babies

Babies can be members of the band, too. If they are around six months old, they may enjoy tapping two spoons together as they are pushed around in their strollers. If they are younger, they will enjoy watching their friends march and listening to them play.

Toddlers

You or an older child can show toddlers how to march.
Encourage them to lift their knees up high while they play
drums or maracas.

Preschoolers

Do you have flags preschoolers can wave in time with the
marching band? If not, they can create quick-and-easy flags by
tying old T-shirts around the end of sticks.

School-Age Children

School-age children probably know more songs than younger
children. Have them share a tune to march to, like "London
Bridge," or call out a made-up title for a song they can create
together with their instruments. They can lead the band, using
sticks as batons to help keep the tempo.

Host Tip

For additional ideas for making homemade instruments for
your marching band, see "Shake It" (page 80) and "Ring Those
Bells" (page 117) in the Music & Movement chapter.

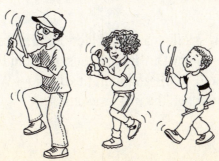

Green, Yellow, Red Lights

The kids will be revving their engines and shifting gears during this backyard game.

What You'll Need	All Ages	Babies	Toddlers	Preschoolers	School-Age Children
Moving bodies!	✋				
Strollers		✋			

Go out to the yard and explain the rules to the children: You will be the traffic light, and they will be the drivers. Designate a road, such as around the perimeter of the yard or from one end of the driveway to the other. Begin by saying, "Green light," which means the drivers must take off (that is, run) along the road. When you say, "Yellow light," they must drive slowly, preparing to stop. But when you say, "Red light," the drivers must freeze. If a driver takes one step after a red light is called, he gets a ticket. The first ticket is a "warning," and the second ticket requires the driver to sit out until the next game. Continue the game until one driver remains on the road.

Babies

Fasten babies in strollers and let older children carefully drive them around for a few thrilling rounds! Or hold them in your arms and let them be the traffic light with you. Watching their friends run around will be just as exciting.

Toddlers

Take a few extra minutes to teach toddlers about the meaning of green, yellow, and red lights, so they can follow along during the game. You or older children may need to prompt them to run quickly, slow down, and stop until they get the hang of it.

Preschoolers

Preschoolers will love to make engines rumble and brakes screech as they drive. They may get caught up in driving, so make sure they understand that a yellow light is a warning that a stop is coming very soon. Can they stop quickly enough?

School-Age Children

For fun, school-age children can drive in reverse: Have them run backward down the road! Just tell them to look out for their friends traveling in the other direction.

Sunflower, Shine for Me

Teach children the joy of planting a flower and watching it grow!

What You'll Need	All Ages	Babies	Toddlers	Preschoolers	School-Age Children
Sunflower seeds				🖐	🖐
Nesting cups		🖐			
Watering cans	🖐				
Hand shovels			🖐	🖐	🖐
Small pots			🖐		
Rocks			🖐		
Journal or camera				🖐	🖐

When there's no longer danger of frost, pick a sunny, open area in your yard. The children can have fun learning how to plant and tend to sunflowers. *Note:* Sunflower seeds are choking hazards. Keep them out of babies' and toddlers' reach during this activity.

Babies

If the babies are around six months old, let them play with their own "pots" (nesting cups, small plastic bowls, or plastic cups) while older friends plant. If you have other flowers in the yard, hold the babies close to them and show them how to sniff their aroma. If the babies are younger, set them in bouncy seats near the other kids. They'll enjoy the smell of freshly dug soil and will especially love watching water cascade from watering cans.

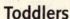

Toddlers

While the older children plant the sunflower seeds, have toddlers practice planting. Give them hand shovels and pots, then let them fill them with soil. Show them how to pat down the soil to level it. They can then dig a small hole, plant a small rock, and pour water on it. If you like, fill small watering cans and ask toddlers to water any flowers in the yard.

Preschoolers and School-Age Children

Preschoolers and school-age children can plant sunflower seeds. Help them dig holes about half-inch deep and one foot apart, drop the seeds in the holes, then pat the soil down. These fast-growing seeds will require full sun exposure and a lot of water. Most sunflowers will grow to maturity within three to six months. Encourage the older children to monitor their sunflowers' growth. Perhaps they can record their observations in a journal or take photos of the sunflowers as they grow. During each visit (at least a few times a week), they can fill up watering cans and make sure the flowers have plenty of water.

Host Tip

In the fall, sunflowers produce seeds you and the older children can eat. Here's how to prepare the seeds:

1. Cut off a ripened sunflower head and push out the seeds.
2. Spread the seeds in a single layer on a baking sheet and, if you wish, sprinkle them lightly with salt.
3. Toast them in a 350°F oven for about ten minutes.

4. Watch the seeds closely to make sure they don't burn.
5. Let them cool before you open the shells and eat the seeds.

Did You Know?
Sunflowers rotate their faces toward the sun as it passes over during the day.

Paws and Claws

Head out on a winter day to look for animal tracks in the snow.

What You'll Need	All Ages	Babies	Toddlers	Preschoolers	School-Age Children
Warm clothes	✋				
Regional guide to animal tracks	✋				
Notebooks and pencils					✋

Make sure children are dressed warmly for this winter excursion. You also may want to wrap babies in fleece blankets. Before heading outdoors, talk to the children about the animals that visit your yard during the winter months. Tell them that each visiting animal leaves tracks, or prints, of

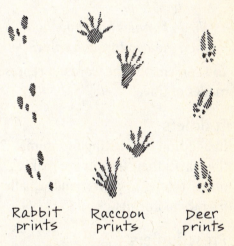

Rabbit prints

Raccoon prints

Deer prints

its paws, feet, or hooves. Here are the tracks of animals common in many snowy parts of North America. You can find others in a regional guide to animal tracks.

Babies

Babies will love the feeling of being bundled up cozy and warm while walking out in the snow. When you come upon some tracks, crouch down and point them out. Even if they can't quite see the tracks, they'll love studying the snow as intently as the other kids do. For fun, make up a song to the tune of "Mary Had a Little Lamb":

Oh, do bunnies hop, hop, hop,
hop, hop, hop,
hop, hop, hop?
Oh, do bunnies hop, hop, hop
when they go through snow?

You can change the words to represent other animals and their modes of travel.

Toddlers

In addition to scouting for animal tracks, ask toddlers about the tracks their friends are making. Do they know which footprints belong to each friend? Challenge them to walk in a friend's footprints.

Preschoolers

Once preschoolers spot animal tracks, encourage them to take a closer look so they can describe them to their friends. Ask them questions, such as, "Is it a small or large track? Are there claw marks or other special patterns?" Preschoolers will appreciate their important detective roles.

School-Age Children
Have school-age children bring along notebooks and pencils to
sketch the tracks. They can later compare the sketches to the
illustrations on page 139 or to regional animal guides. You
may also want to check out websites such as http://www.bear-
tracker.com for more information.

Host Tip
The night before this activity, you may want to leave apple
pieces someplace in the yard. This may coax the animals to
visit the yard and leave lots of tracks!

Won't Knock Us Down

This bottle game will be a knockout success!

What You'll Need	All Ages	Babies	Toddlers	Preschoolers	School-Age Children
Empty water bottles (with a little bit of sand on the bottom to weigh them down)	✋				
Foam balls	✋				

Set up a number of bottles side by side in a line on a flat outdoor surface. Select one child to serve as a catcher who will stand behind the formation, retrieve the ball, and roll it back to the player. Everyone gets three tries each turn to roll a foam ball and knock down as many bottles as possible.

Babies

If babies are crawling or walking with support, let them try to knock down the bottles. Set them in front of the bottles and let them make their way toward them. Cheer when they knock a few down. If they need motivation to aim for the bottles, let them watch older friends take turns knocking the bottles down with the ball. It won't take the babies long to figure out the goal of the game! If the babies aren't mobile yet, hold them in your lap near the bottles so they can reach out and swat them down. Guide their hands if they need help.

Toddlers

Toddlers can stand close to the bottles when it's their turn. They may be more apt to drop the balls into a roll, but try teaching them to sit the balls on the ground and then push the ball away instead.

Preschoolers

Have preschoolers take three giant steps back from the bottles before they roll the ball. After each turn, they should move three additional steps further. Encourage them to experiment with ways to line up and roll their balls accurately. Once they perfect their aim, they can try to knock down bottles with their eyes closed.

School-Age Children

Chances are school-age children will have more power than younger children. They will need to stand a good distance away when rolling. For an extra challenge, let their friends space the bottles farther apart in the line. This way, the bottles will be less likely to strike each other and fall down like dominoes. School-age children will have to aim carefully at specific spots in the line to knock as many down as they can in three tries.

Water "Painting"

Unlike real painting projects, this water activity will never make a mess!

What You'll Need	All Ages	Babies	Toddlers	Preschoolers	School-Age Children
Buckets	🖐				
Various paintbrushes	🖐				
Chalk				🖐	
Watch				🖐	

On a warm day, send the kids outside with a few buckets of water and clean paintbrushes. Let them "paint" the side of the house, the steps, the driveway, or outdoor toys with the water. They'll enjoy giving the objects a nice sheen.

Babies

Brush the babies' feet with a bit of water. Creep the brush up their legs and then back down to their toes. They'll enjoy the sensation, especially if they're ticklish!

Toddlers

Encourage toddlers to paint objects both high (like a wall) and low (like a driveway). Stretching and squatting will strengthen their major muscle groups. Give them bigger paintbrushes, which might be easier for them to handle.

Preschoolers

Ask preschoolers to predict how much pavement they can paint in one minute. Mark their goals with chalk, then challenge them to make the predictions come true. Keep track of the time on your watch, and cheer them on! See if they can paint bigger areas next time.

School-Age Children

Have school-age children write secret, evaporating messages with paintbrushes, then have others read them. Can they read them before the messages evaporate? They'll have to be quick! Encourage school-age children to use different paintbrushes, different amounts of water, and different "canvases" to see how long they can make the messages last. Write messages for them, too!

Watching the Clouds Pass

Children's imaginations will soar as they watch clouds.

What You'll Need	All Ages	Babies	Toddlers	Preschoolers	School-Age Children
Blanket	✋				
Cotton balls		✋			

Relax on a blanket on a mostly sunny day and watch the clouds float by. Have the children use their imaginations to describe the shapes the clouds make. This activity is also great during a car ride. If anyone needs a distraction or entertainment, let the clouds help you out!

Babies

Lay babies on their backs and point out the clouds to them. Show them how the clouds move by blowing gently on their faces. They'll love the sensation. If you like, let the babies feel a "cloud" by rubbing a cotton ball on their hands or cheeks.

Toddlers

Depending on the toddlers' vocabulary, they may suggest a cloud looks like a simple object, such as a circle, or a favorite object, such as a dog or truck. Have them lie on their back and try touching the cloud with their toes, elbows, hands, and even their noses. This is a great way to have busy toddlers focus on the clouds for a little while!

Preschoolers

Name a category, such as animals, letters, or cars, and ask preschoolers to point out clouds that look like something from that group. For instance, if you say, "Animal," they may see a cloud that looks like a dog.

School-Age Children

School-age children's abilities to see detailed images in the clouds may amaze you. Let them tell stories about the things they see in the sky, incorporating several cloud formations. As the clouds change and shift, their stories will, too.

Host Tip

Back inside, the children can re-create the clouds they saw using blue construction paper and cotton balls.

Did You Know?

In 1802, a scientist named Luke Howard classified clouds into three different groups: cumulus (puffy clouds), cirrus (wispy clouds), and stratus (clouds that blanket the sky).

Letterboxing

Letterboxing is a fun pastime that uses navigational skills to find hidden treasures in outdoor public places. The kids will love the hunt!

What You'll Need	All Ages	Babies	Toddlers	Preschoolers	School-Age Children
Stamps and ink pad (or carve a stamp from an eraser)	✋				
Notebook or journal and pen	✋				
Computer with Internet access and printer	✋				

Explain to the children that you'll be going on a search for a letterbox—a special container someone has hidden in your area. When you find it, you'll leave a stamp in its logbook, plus make one in your own logbook. Here are the steps to get started on your first letterbox hunt:

1. Think up a "trail name" with the children. This will be your letterboxing identity. You may want to use your real name, but most letterboxers use a nickname or a name with special meaning.

2. Find a small rubber stamp and ink pad. Like your trail name, the stamp should represent something special about you. You may wish to buy a special stamp beforehand or make a homemade stamp by carving a special symbol into a large eraser. You can have one stamp for the team, or

multiple stamps, so the kids can then use them with their own families.

3. Find a small notebook or blank journal to use as a logbook to record your finds. Don't forget to bring a pen, too.

4. Visit http://www.letterboxing.org to find lists of clues to letterboxes hidden in your area. According to the site, there are about twenty thousand letterboxes hidden in North America alone. Older children may enjoy looking up clues with your supervision. When you've decided on a letterbox to find, print the clues.

5. Gather your gear and your team of hunters—it's time to head out! When at the site, encourage the children to follow the printed-out clues to find the letterbox. Remind them that letterboxing is an environmentally friendly activity; they should not dig, trample vegetation, or disturb wildlife during the hunt. When they've found the box, help them mark its logbook with your stamp, write the name of your city, and date and sign it with your trail name. Remind kids to record the find in their logbook using the stamp found in the letterbox.

Babies

Strap babies into carriers so they can feel like real participants on this hunt. Share the sense of adventure with them as you make your way to the hiding spot. With great animation, describe all the sights and sounds or sing silly parodies like, "Over the walkway and through the field, a-hunting we will go!"

Toddlers

Toddlers will enjoy exploring with their friends, especially if you end up in fun places like parks and playgrounds. Give them the special task of carrying the stamps in their pockets. They can also be the ones to stamp the logbooks found in the letterboxes.

Preschoolers

Once you find the letterbox, put preschoolers in charge of opening up the logbooks and marking them with the stamps from the letterboxes. Ask them if they'd like you to add any additional notes to logbooks about the search.

School-Age Children

School-age children should be the keepers of the clues. They can read each step out loud and offer instructions on which way to go next. They can also be in charge of recording your trail name, city, and the date next to your stamp in the letterbox's logbook. They could also add a few comments on the hiding space or the weather.

I took my son and nephew on this adventure, and they loved it! It gave them a great sense of accomplishment when they found the letterbox.

—Lisa

Raking 'Em Up

Turn the chore of raking leaves into a fun activity!

What You'll Need	All Ages	Babies	Toddlers	Preschoolers	School-Age Children
Rakes			🖐	🖐	🖐
Blanket		🖐			
Stick				🖐	🖐

Head outside on an autumn day. Rake some leaves into a pile and let the kids have fun in it!

Babies

Lay babies on a blanket. Have older friends show them a few vibrantly colored leaves and drop a few gently over their bodies. Babies six months or older can sit by a small pile of leaves and crunch them in their hands as you recite this poem:

Leaves orange, yellow, red.
"Crunch! Crunch!
Crunch! Crunch!"
That's what the leaves said.

Toddlers

Jumping takes a lot of coordination. Help toddlers jump into the pile by holding their hands and jumping with them. You can also kneel in front of them, hold them under their arms, and lift them up when they jump.

Preschoolers and School-Age Children

Preschoolers and school-age children have the body strength to rake. Have them work together to rake some leaves into a nice-size pile to test their jumping skills. Place a stick about two feet away from the pile. Have them begin on the other side of the stick and try jumping into the pile of leaves. Did they reach the pile? Sing this song to give them the go-ahead to jump:

[Children's names] be nimble,
[children's names] run a mile,
[children's names] jump into the leaf pile!

If they hit the pile the first time, move the stick back another foot. Can they do it again?

Sprinkler Race

This sprinkler game will get kids soaked and satisfied on a
warm day!

What You'll Need	All Ages	Babies	Toddlers	Preschoolers	School-Age Children
Sprinkler	🖐				
Bucket			🖐	🖐	🖐
Plastic cups	🖐				
Watch			🖐	🖐	🖐

Set up a sprinkler and place a bucket a reasonable distance
from it. Give toddlers, preschoolers, and school-age children
plastic cups and instruct them to use them to "collect" water
from the sprinkler. The object of the game is to work as a team
to transfer as much water as they can from their cups to the
bucket within one minute. Depending on their strategy—and
your sprinkler style—they can fill their cups simultaneously or
do it as a relay. When one minute is up, tell them to stop and
see how full the bucket is. Dump the water (use it to water the
flowers or trees), then have them try to beat their amount.

Babies

As older children run this race, hold babies near the sprinkler's
stream so they can feel the cool mist on their bodies and faces.
Fill cups with water and let them dip their hands into it.

Toddlers

Pouring the water into the bucket will be toddlers' favorite part, so they may not let their cups fill for very long before running off to empty them. Let them enjoy the game in this way. Running back and forth is good for their legs, and pouring the water is good for their dexterity!

Preschoolers

Challenge preschoolers to figure out how to get the most water into their cups in the fastest amount of time. Where do they need to stand? How do they need to hold their cups? When they have good strategies, have them share them with their teammates.

School-Age Children

School-age children will likely enjoy splashing around, but you can also use this activity to introduce math concepts like fractions and whole numbers. Ask them to predict how long it would take to fill the whole bucket. To do this, have them determine what fraction of the bucket they fill in one minute. Then help them use that fraction to predict how many more minutes it would take to fill the whole bucket. Have them inform the team that in the next round, they'll test their predictions.

Our Own Terrariums

Children can collect some outdoor specimens in their own tiny terrariums.

What You'll Need	All Ages	Babies	Toddlers	Preschoolers	School-Age Children
Plastic jars			🖐	🖐	🖐
Plastic water bottle		🖐			
Hand shovels	🖐				
Rocks, soil, leaves, and twigs	🖐				
Small plastic animals or insects (or real bugs)	🖐				
Screwdriver or scissors				🖐	🖐

A terrarium is a container, usually enclosed, for observing and researching animals or plants. Each child can easily make a terrarium by washing out a clear, deep, plastic jar. When the jars are dry, go to your yard or a nearby park with the kids. Have them cover the bottom of their jars with rocks. Next, have them use a hand shovel to add a layer of soil over the rocks, then place leaves and twigs on top of the soil. Back home, give each child a small plastic animal or insect toy to place on top of the leaves and twigs. Have them cover their jars and use their imaginations to note what's happening in the terrariums! Older children may want real bugs instead (see next page).

Babies

Make terrariums for babies with an empty water bottle instead of a jar. Secure the top on the bottle. If babies are six months or older, let them hold or even shake their terrariums. If they are younger, hold the bottle close to them so they can see what's inside.

Toddlers

Help toddlers gather rocks and leaves for their terrariums. As you help place items into the jars, count the number of leaves, rocks, and twigs out loud. Encourage them to count with you.

Preschoolers and School-Age Children

Instead of adding plastic toys, preschoolers and school-age children may prefer to add live insects like caterpillars or ants to their terrariums. Make sure to punch air holes in the lids using a screwdriver or scissors, and have children toss in fresh leaves for food. Encourage them to handle the terrariums gently and note all they can about their insects before releasing them at the end of the activity.

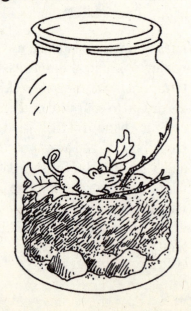

Twig-and-Rock Houses

Build model homes using twigs, rocks, or other natural materials.

What You'll Need	All Ages	Babies	Toddlers	Preschoolers	School-Age Children
Natural materials, such as rocks, twigs, leaves, and so on	🖐				

Head to your yard or nearby park with the children and help them collect twigs, rocks, or other natural materials. Have them sit in a flat, open space on grass or dirt, and then encourage them to use the materials to build houses. Children can use their imaginations to construct the houses, or here are some building suggestions:

Rock House
Press long, flat rocks upright and side by side into the ground, and balance other rocks horizontally across the tops. Or simply make a rock pile in the shape of a house.

Twig House
Push similar-size twigs upright and side by side into the ground. Build four walls, then lay twigs horizontally across the top to create the roof.

Twig Tepee
Lean twigs upright against one another.

Babies

Babies can create leaf "houses." Hold the baby in your lap as you pile leaves in mounds in front of you both. The baby may have just as much fun destroying the house as building it!

Toddlers

To make houses, toddlers may enjoy simply lining up twigs and rocks or placing them on top of one another in a pile. For added fun, decorate the houses' "yards" by arranging rocks and twigs to make the first letter in the toddlers' names.

Preschoolers

Preschoolers have experiences with building blocks, but building with rocks and twigs will challenge them. Encourage them to combine some water and dirt to make mud that will better secure their building materials.

School-Age Children

This project is perfect for school-age children because it provides many levels of challenge. Their houses can be intricately small or quite large and sprawling. Have them collect other nature items, such as pine needles, acorns, or flower petals, to decorate their houses or add some extensions, such as a walkway.

Host Tip

If the area permits, have the children build their homes close together to create a model neighborhood.

Up, Up, Paper Airplane

Help children create and fly their own paper airplanes.

What You'll Need	All Ages	Babies	Toddlers	Preschoolers	School-Age Children
Construction paper			✋	✋	✋
Rocks				✋	✋
Marker				✋	✋
Sticks				✋	✋

Children will love making paper airplanes as much as flying them. To make a basic paper airplane, follow these directions. You'll need to make airplanes for toddlers, but older children should be able to make their own with a little help.

1. Place a sheet of construction paper in front of you so the short sides are horizontal and the long sides are vertical.
2. Fold down the top two corners to meet. This creates two triangle flaps.
3. Fold the paper in half so the triangle flaps come together. This will create a point.
4. Position the paper so the point faces to your left, the open edges are at the top, and the creased edge is at the bottom.
5. Fold down the top layer's edge to meet the bottom crease.
6. Flip the paper over so the triangle point faces to your right, then repeat Step 5.
7. Pick up the paper from the long edge with one hand, and use the other hand to unfold the side flaps 90 degrees to create wings.

Babies

While older children make and fly their paper airplanes, hold babies and fly them like an airplane. For babies younger than four months, hold them face-up and use one hand to support their heads and necks and the other hand to support their bottoms. Gently sway them about six inches from your body. For older babies, you can hold them face-down, using one hand to support their chest and wrapping the other arm around their hips. If you like, sing the following song to the tune of "Mary Had a Little Lamb" as you fly:

We are flying on a plane,
on a plane,
on a plane.
We are flying on a plane,
way up here in the sky!

Toddlers

Make paper airplanes for toddlers and show them how to fly them. They may need time to figure out how to release the paper airplanes properly. Regardless, applaud their efforts! If they become frustrated, encourage them to fly their airplanes by holding them high while zooming around the yard.

Preschoolers and School-Age Children

Encourage preschoolers and school-age children to make their own paper airplanes. Help them when needed. They may need to make several practice airplanes before getting it right, so have several sheets of paper on hand. Here are some games they can play with their paper airplanes:

Aim Practice

Collect five small rocks and number them 1 through 5 with a marker. The numbers represent points. Place the rocks in random order a few feet away from a starting point. Have children stand at the starting point and throw their airplanes toward the rocks. When they land, note the rock each is nearest. The number on the respective rock is the number of points that child earns. Continue to play until one child earns ten points.

Plane Landing

Use two sticks to create a start line and a finish line a few feet apart. Have children throw their airplanes from the start line toward the finish line. Wherever the planes land, children must collect them and throw them again from that spot. Have them continue until one of them flies a plane across the finish line.

Up and Away

Have children fly their airplanes into the air and count how long each one stays afloat. Whose flies the longest?

Host Tip

For more paper airplane fun, we recommend *The World Record Paper Airplane Book* by Ken Blackburn and Jeff Lammers. Blackburn holds the world record for the longest recorded paper airplane flight, lasting 27.6 seconds.

Beanbag Race

Use homemade beanbags to run this fun race.

What You'll Need	All Ages	Babies	Toddlers	Preschoolers	School-Age Children
Large socks in different colors	🖐				
Dried beans	🖐				
Rubber bands	🖐				
Long and short sticks	🖐				

Help children fill large socks with dried beans. Try to give each child a different-colored sock. Tightly close the socks with rubber bands. Then head outside to a fairly flat grassy area with the beanbags. Make a starting line with a long stick and have the kids stand behind it. On the count of three, have children toss their beanbags as far as they can in front of them. After the bags have landed, have children race to collect them and return to the starting line. The first child to cross the starting line wins. Race again as often as the kids want. If they like, have them forgo the race and just have fun with the beanbags as described below.

Babies

A beanbag will delight babies' senses. Rub the socks up and down their bodies and along their cheeks, letting the beans massage them. If they can grasp objects, give them the bean-bags and let them strengthen their finger muscles as they feel the beans. If babies are beginning to show signs of standing and walking, they can "run" the beanbag race, too! Help them toss their beanbags, then support them under their arms while they try to walk and collect the beanbags. (Caution: Beans pose a choking hazard for babies and toddlers, so make sure all beanbags are securely closed!)

Toddlers
Because toddlers are learning to hold and release objects, it may be easier for them to toss their beanbags upward than forward. Encourage them to throw the bags as many times as needed to get it to a designated spot a short distance from the start line.

Preschoolers
Tossing beanbags will strengthen preschoolers' large-motor skills. Encourage them to throw their beanbags overhand, underhand, and backwards over their shoulders. Can they think of other ways to toss it? Which way lets them toss the bag the farthest?

School-Age Children
School-age children can track their beanbag tosses by marking where each attempt lands with a short stick. Encourage them to beat their best tosses. For a more-physical challenge, tell them to hop to retrieve the beanbags and skip back to the start line. Their younger friends may try to mimic those actions!

Hop with Me

This classic sidewalk game is sure to get the whole group hopping!

What You'll Need	All Ages	Babies	Toddlers	Preschoolers	School-Age Children
Chalk	🖐				
Small rocks				🖐	🖐
Beanbag (see page 162 for a homemade variety)			🖐		

On a sidewalk or driveway, help older children draw a chalk hopscotch court with ten connecting boxes like so:

1. Begin by drawing Box 1.
2. Draw two boxes side by side centered over Box 1, and number them 2 and 3.
3. Move up and draw Box 4 centered over Boxes 2 and 3.
4. Draw Boxes 5 and 6 side by side centered over Box 4.
5. Move up and draw Box 7 centered over Boxes 5 and 6.
6. Draw Boxes 8 and 9 side by side centered over Box 7.
7. Lastly, move up and draw Box 10 centered over Boxes 8 and 9.

Teach children how to play traditional hopscotch: For each player's first turn, they must toss a small rock onto the first square on the court, and then hop through the court without landing on the first square. When landing on the single boxes, the players must hop on one foot. When landing on the side-by-side boxes, they must straddle the boxes with one foot on each. On the way back through the court, they must stop and pick up their rocks before continuing on. On the second turn, the players must toss the rock onto the second square, and so on with each round. If a player's rock misses a box, or if the player loses her balance or steps on a line, her turn is over. With her next turn, a player picks up where she left off.

Encourage children to play the traditional form of hopscotch or the following age-appropriate variations:

Babies

If babies are around six months or older, hold them up so they can "walk" their way through the hopscotch court. If you like, bounce them slightly as you move along. Hold younger babies in your arms and gently bounce along the hopscotch court. They'll love the fun movement.

Toddlers

Hold toddlers' hands and walk through the hopscotch court as you count the number in each square out loud. Instead of a rock, give them a beanbag to toss onto the court (so there's less danger if they lose control of their aim), and see if they can name the number it lands on. Have them retrieve the bags and toss them again. If they like, let them bounce or hop through the court however they wish.

Preschoolers

At this age, preschoolers may not have mastered hopping on one foot, so challenge them to give it a try through the hopscotch court. If they have trouble hopping the entire court on one foot, let them jump with two feet.

School-Age Children

Once school-age children have mastered the traditional hop-scotch court, have them try another version called Snail. In this variation, draw the court to look like a snail shell (see the illustration below). Have the children choose one foot to hop on to reach the center. They can hop only once in each square and can't hop on any lines. If they hop in a square more than once or hop on any lines, they'll have to start over.

Did You Know?

Hopscotch began in ancient Britain during the rule of the Roman Empire. The original hopscotch courts were over one hundred feet long and used for military training exercises.

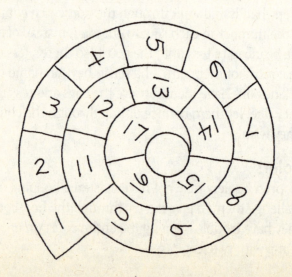

Chapter 5

Out & About

Ah, the car ride: the whining kids, the bathroom emergencies, the two-minute errands that end up taking two hours...

—Lisa

We know you've got places to go—and we know you often have other kids along with your own (friends, carpools, family). But who says you all can't enjoy the ride? This chapter holds true to the belief that life happens during the journey. Here you'll find simple, creative ideas to have fun out and about, such as when you're riding in a car, sitting in a restaurant, or waiting in a checkout line. And because you're on the go, most of these activities require only your imaginations!

Freeze!

Here's a fun, easy way to entertain children while in the car, a waiting room, or anywhere else that requires patience.

What You'll Need	All Ages	Babies	Toddlers	Preschoolers	School-Age Children
Your hands and some imagination!	🖐				

To begin the game, start clapping a steady rhythm. (If your hands aren't free, say, "Chug, Chug," in rhythm while the children clap.) Ask the children to join in. After a moment or so, say, "Freeze!" and stay completely still and quiet. The children will follow the command, but they'll eventually start giggling! Have the children take turns leading the clapping and saying, "Freeze!" If you're someplace where clapping isn't appropriate (for example, in a quiet waiting room), do a silent action, like patting your belly or making a goofy face.

Babies

If babies are six months or older, they may join in as they clap. Encourage older children to praise babies (and toddlers) for their efforts! Older children can gently help younger babies clap their hands until someone says, "Freeze!" The babies will love the rhythm and movement.

Toddlers

Toddlers will enjoy anticipating the command to freeze, but they may have trouble following it. To help them focus on the command, use a nearby object as a visual cue. This object can be a crayon, toy, sippy cup, or other handy object (including your own hand). Tell toddlers that when the leader says, "Freeze!" and holds up the object, they must stay still until the object is lowered.

Preschoolers
Many preschoolers love to be goofy. When it's preschoolers' turn to lead the clapping, have them make silly noises to accompany their actions. If noise isn't appropriate where you are, suggest that they make a silly face instead. When it's time to freeze, regaining their composure may be a challenge, so encourage their efforts.

School-Age Children
Along with clapping, school-age children may want to challenge their friends with other actions. For example, they may put their hands on their knees or touch their nose between each clap. When they give the command to freeze, they may challenge their friends to not just stay still, but to also close their eyes or fold their hands.

> My eight-month-old son learned to clap during one of these games. He loved copying the movements of his older brother.
> —Lisa

Table Memory

While waiting at a restaurant, keep kids busy with this fun memory game.

What You'll Need	All Ages	Babies	Toddlers	Preschoolers	School-Age Children
Items on the restaurant table, including menus, creamer packets, sugar packets, napkins, utensils, condiment bottles, and so on	✋				

While sitting at a restaurant table, place three different items in front of you. Ask children to identify them, then have them close their eyes. Move one item to your lap. Have them open their eyes and tell you which item is missing. The children can then take turns hiding an item and challenging the others' memories.

Babies

Babies may be too young to play this memory game, but they can play another type of memory game: peekaboo! Peekaboo strengthens their sense of object permanence (the understanding that something exists even when not in sight). Encourage the older children to play peekaboo with the babies using a napkin, the menu, or another item.

Toddlers

After you hide an item in your lap, toddlers may not be as quick as the older children to identify it. To give toddlers a chance to test their memory, encourage older kids to let them identify the missing item at least once. When it's a toddler's turn to hide an item, have older kids close their eyes while you prompt the toddler to hide an item in his lap.

Preschoolers

To further challenge preschoolers' memory, rearrange the order of the items after hiding one. After they correctly identify the missing item, ask them to put the other items in their original order. When preschoolers hide an item, encourage them to give their friends a hint that describes the missing item. For example, they may say, "I took away something red."

School-Age Children

Challenge school-age children to pay close attention to detail. After they correctly identify a missing item, ask them a more-detailed question about it, such as, "What color is the label on the ketchup bottle?" or, "What kind of jelly is in the packet?"

Host Tip
If there aren't enough items on the table for this game, use items from your diaper bag, purse, or wallet.

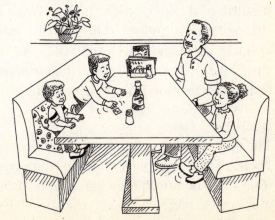

These Little Kids Went to the Market

Here's a fun way to make grocery shopping a team effort!

What You'll Need	All Ages	Babies	Toddlers	Preschoolers	School-Age Children
Supermarket flyers or magazines	✋				
Child-safe scissors	✋				
Index cards	✋				
Glue sticks	✋				
Crayons	✋				

Before your next trip to the supermarket, tell older children a few items from your grocery list. They can cut out pictures of those items from supermarket flyers or magazines, then glue the pictures onto separate index cards. Or they can draw pictures of the items with crayons. When it's time to go to the supermarket, give toddlers, preschoolers, and school-age children each a few cards and ask them, "What's the food on your card?" After they've identified the item, say, "Your job is to look for this food as we shop. Will you help me do that?"

Babies

The grocery store is full of educational opportunities for babies. Encourage older children to show and describe the items they find from their cards to the babies. For example,

"This is a red, crunchy apple." Babies will enjoy the colors, smells, and interaction.

Toddlers

When you get close to an item on the toddlers' cards, prompt them by saying, "Do you see the yellow bananas? They are very close now." When they identify the item, let them hold it and examine it. Talk to them about each item, such as, "These bananas are smooth and yellow." This will support their growing vocabulary.

Preschoolers and School-Age Children

In addition to creating cards for everyday items on your grocery list, preschoolers and school-age children may enjoy making cards for ingredients in a favorite dish or meal. For example, tell them that this week you will make tacos. Ask them to help you determine what items you need to buy for the meal, and have them create cards for those items. At the store, give them the cards so they can collect the ingredients for this special meal.

Host Tip

Create cards of items you buy often (for example, bread, eggs, milk, bananas, and so on) and use them every time you visit the supermarket with children.

Diddle, Diddle, Doo

While riding in the car with children, recite this knee-slapping, silly rhyme that talks about important people in your community.

What You'll Need	All Ages	Babies	Toddlers	Preschoolers	School-Age Children
Hands and knees!	✋				

As you teach kids the rhyme, show them how to slap each hand on each knee at the same time in rhythm. (If you're driving, wait until a stoplight so your hands are free to demonstrate the slaps.) Once they have the rhythm down, lead them with this rhyme:

Hey, diddle, diddle,
who's in the middle
when you're feeling sick?
A doctor, that's who!
Diddle, diddle, doo.
GO DOCTOR!

Hey, diddle, diddle,
who's in the middle
when there is a fire?
A firefighter, that's who!
Diddle, diddle, doo.
GO FIREFIGHTER!

Hey, diddle, diddle,
who's in the middle
when you need the mail?
A mailcarrier, that's who!
Diddle, diddle, doo.
GO MAILCARRIER!

Hey, diddle, diddle,
who's in the middle
when you want to learn?
A teacher, that's who!
Diddle, diddle, doo.
GO TEACHER!

Babies and Toddlers

Babies and toddlers will enjoy listening to everyone recite this rhyme and slap their knees. They may even try to slap their own knees! If you like, help toddlers make the connection between the people described in the rhyme and the people they know. For example, after reciting the verse about the doctor, say to the toddlers, "A doctor is someone who makes you feel all better. Dr. Jones is your doctor. You know who she is, don't you?"

Preschoolers and School-Age Children

Encourage preschoolers and school-age children to come up with more people in the community to add to the rhyme, like a police officer, librarian, or garbage collector. When they've finished reciting the rhyme, ask the children what they think of each person's job. Does it sound fun, easy, or hard? This exercise may get them thinking about what they want to be when they grow up.

> This activity is my family's favorite during car trips.
> —Lisa

Where Is Everyone Going?

With imagination and storytelling, car rides are entertaining! During your next car ride, let older children take turns telling a tale about the people in a nearby car.

What You'll Need	All Ages	Babies	Toddlers	Preschoolers	School-Age Children
Imagination!	✋				

Babies

Although babies are too young to tell a story, they will enjoy listening to one told by a loved one. They may even coo and smile as a way to interact with their friends when they hear their happy voices and see their smiles as they tell stories. Babies' friends can nurture the babies' own "storytelling" skills by responding to their babbles with questions like, "And then what happened?"

Toddlers

As toddlers listen to tales, they may join in when they hear words they recognize. For instance, if the storyteller says, "That man in the car looks like Papa," toddlers may look to see for themselves and yell, "Papa!" Let them get involved in this way—it shows their listening skills are developing! If you like, have older children further involve toddlers in the storytelling by asking them questions such as, "Where is that car going?"

Preschoolers and School-Age Children

To help preschoolers and school-age children begin their stories, ask a few leading questions, such as, "Who do you think is in the car ahead of us? Where do you think they're going? What are they going to do there?" Encourage children to use their imaginations to answer these questions and spin a tale! School-age children may not need these questions to start their story; in that case, say simply, "Tell me about the people traveling behind us."

I love doing this activity with my children. My pre-schooler inevitably drops a hint about where he wishes he were headed. For example, he'll say, "I think that man is going to the ice-cream store because he is SO hungry for ice cream!"

—Heather

ABC Games

These alphabet games are fun ways to pass time while waiting with children in a doctor's office, a checkout line, or another place that requires patience.

What You'll Need	All Ages	Babies	Toddlers	Preschoolers	School-Age Children
Scrap paper				✋	
Pencil				✋	

Babies

Use each baby's first name in a cheer with their friends. Babies will love to hear their friends cheer for them! For example:

You: "Give me an *A*!"

Children: "*A*!"

You: "Give me a *D*!"

Children: "*D*!"

You: "Give me an *A*!"

Children: "*A*!"

You: "Give me an *M*!"

Children: "*M*!"

You: "What's that spell?"

Children: "ADAM!"

Toddlers

Show toddlers a highly visible, large letter, such as one in a magazine title. Say the letter several times, then ask them to repeat it. To use toddlers' sense of touch to help remember the formation of the letter, have them trace the letters with their fingers. If they can't reach the letter, use your finger to draw it on the back of their hands.

Preschoolers

If preschoolers know how to spell their names, challenge them to find each letter somewhere around them. Then encourage them to find the letters in other words they know how to spell. If preschoolers don't know how to spell their names or other words, print the words on scrap paper and have them find each letter around them.

School-Age Children

Have school-age children locate each letter of the alphabet somewhere around them. They must find each letter in order, which means they must find an *A* before finding a *B* and so on. They may need to say, "Pass," for hard-to-find letters. If you like, keep track of the time it takes them to find the letters and have them repeat the activity to see whether they can beat that time.

Ten Things

This fun counting game will keep children's attention when you're out and about.

What You'll Need	All Ages	Babies	Toddlers	Preschoolers	School-Age Children
Paper and pen				✋	✋

To play, pose a question that requires ten answers. For example, point to a car ahead of you and say, "I wonder what that family likes to eat for dinner. Can we come up with ten things you think they like to eat?" Here are other ideas for questions:

- "Can you name ten things that truck driver may have in his truck?"
- "Can you name ten kinds of fruit?"
- "Can you name ten things a baby does before he goes to bed?"
- "Can you name ten things you would find in a trunk?"
- "Can you name ten things you might find in the kitchen of a restaurant?"
- "Can you name ten games that family sitting across from us might play together?"
- "Can you name ten kinds of animals that live in the woods over there?"

Babies

Babies can't contribute answers, but they can still participate. For example, they will love to hear their friends recite the following number rhyme that counts from one to ten:

How much do we love baby?
We love baby—one.
We love baby—one,
because he's so much fun!
How much do we love baby?
We love baby—two.
We love baby—two,
because he loves us, too!

To continue, ask other children to make up rhyming responses for the remaining numbers up to ten.

Toddlers

You can involve toddlers in the activity by asking a question specific to them. For example, ask children for ten things toddlers like to eat. Then ask toddlers, "Do you like to eat bananas?" If they say yes, then they contributed bananas to the list.

Preschoolers and School-Age Children

Older children can likely provide ten answers to every question. To keep track, they can make a mark on a scrap of paper for every answer they give. Make sure they count the toddler's contributions, too! You can also customize the questions to fit their specific interests. For example, if the preschoolers love dinosaurs, ask them to name ten facts about dinosaurs. If the school-age children are currently studying geography at school, ask them to name ten states.

What Do You Hear?

This fun game will have kids sounding like the animals, cars, and other things around them!

What You'll Need	All Ages	Babies	Toddlers	Preschoolers	School-Age Children
Voices!	✋				

When you are out on a walk, in the car, or in a restaurant, ask the children to be quiet for a moment and listen to the sounds around them. What do they hear? Then have each child take a turn using only his voice to imitate something he heard. Everyone else should then try to guess the source of the sound being imitated.

Babies
Babies will enjoy listening to their friends play this game, but they may want to make some noise themselves. If they coo or happily emit a high-pitched squeal, say to the other children, "The baby wants to share, too! What does that sound remind you of?"

Toddlers
By this age, toddlers may know how to make many sounds with their voices, but they may need some direction to play this game. When it's their turn to imitate a sound, privately discuss with them some sounds you've heard in the area. For example, ask them, "Can you hear the big trucks driving by? What sound do

they make?" Otherwise, prompt them to make a particular sound for their turn. For example, say, "What does a cow say?"

Preschoolers and School-Age Children

Preschoolers and school-age children can take separate turns, or for a special challenge, you can encourage them to work together to create a "soundscape" of multiple sources. Have them listen and look around the area for ideas, whisper their plans to each other, then perform the sounds. For instance, if they decide to imitate a dog and its owner, one can bark and the other can say a command like "Heel!"

Chapter 6

Learning & Exploring

Kids learn best from one another. At an early age, I loved learning so much, I recruited neighborhood children to come to my basement for math and art lessons. I had a chalkboard, makeshift desks, and even, for an unlucky few, some homework!

—Lisa

This chapter proves that nearly anything can be an educational experience for children. Whether these activities cultivate a love of reading and writing, inspire the art of storytelling, or experiment with simple science, they'll have kids learning and exploring together. In each one, we provide ideas for creating a "classroom" with simple materials and instructions to challenge and engage children's minds.

Spin the Storybox

Design simple, reusable storyboxes to spark children's storytelling skills.

What You'll Need	All Ages	Babies	Toddlers	Preschoolers	School-Age Children
Old picture books and magazines	✋				
Empty cube-shaped tissue box	✋				
Child-safe scissors and glue	✋				
Index card	✋				
Journal or notebook and pencil					✋

Have children search through magazines to find pictures of animals, people, toys, and other objects that strike their fancy. Decide as a group which six images to cut out. Then create a story box by gluing one picture onto each side of a cube-shaped tissue box. Before gluing a picture to the top of the box, cut and glue an index card to cover the dispensing hole. When the storybox is complete, have children take turns being the storyteller—the one who tosses or rolls the storybox to see which picture lands face-up. The storyteller must then tell a story about the image. Encourage the storytellers to let their imaginations run free when telling the tales.

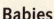

Babies

Although babies can't tell much of a tale, they will love to snuggle up as they watch the colorful storybox and listen to playmates spin stories. When it's baby's turn to be the storyteller, you can make up a tale from his tiny perspective.

Toddlers

Encourage toddler storytellers to identify the picture and talk a little about it. This exercise will strengthen fledgling vocabulary and language skills. For example, you may say, "This is a clock. Can you say 'clock'?" Whatever response the storyteller gives, say, "Yeah! That's right, 'clock'!" Then help create a sentence with the word in it: "The clock says it's noon, and the kids have to come inside for lunch."

Preschoolers

Preschoolers' growing imaginations will let them tell entertaining stories. Encourage them to weave parts of their everyday life into their tale. For example, a preschooler may include her siblings, friends, or preschool in her story. This activity may even provide insight into the preschooler's thoughts or feelings about situations in her daily life. (See Lisa's note on the next page.)

School-Age Children

Challenge school-age children to include the elements of a formal story when telling a tale. They can make sure their story has a setting, different characters, a conflict, a solution, and a closing. After the activity, encourage them to record and perhaps continue their stories in a journal or notebook.

Host Tip

This activity is also a great opportunity to share a story from your childhood. For instance, if the storybox rolls to a picture of a house, you can say, "This picture reminds me of the house I grew up in when I was your age. Would you like to hear about it?"

> Through this activity, I learned about something that had happened at my son's preschool—feelings he was still trying to sort out. My three-year-old used a picture on his storybox to describe two boys fighting over a toy and a teacher taking the toy away.
>
> —Lisa

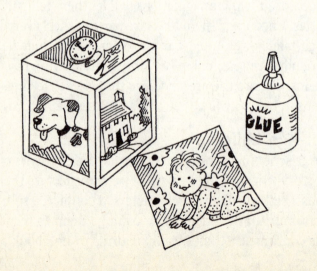

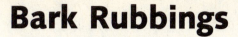

Bark Rubbings

Take children outside to make rubbings of the bark on trees in a yard or neighborhood park.

What You'll Need	All Ages	Babies	Toddlers	Preschoolers	School-Age Children
Paper			👋	👋	👋
Jumbo crayons with wrappers removed			👋	👋	👋
Duct tape			👋	👋	👋
Glue sticks			👋	👋	👋
Stapler			👋	👋	👋
Tree guide			👋	👋	👋
Blanket		👋			
Pen				👋	👋

Before heading out to the yard or the park, give each child a bare jumbo crayon and a sheet of paper. Once outside, have the children select their trees—each a different kind, if possible. Attach each child's paper to the tree with duct tape. Instruct children to firmly rub the length of the crayon up and down the paper to make bark rubbings. Before heading back inside, have them each pick up a leaf that's fallen from their respective trees.

When back inside, help children glue their leaves onto the paper with their bark rubbings. When done, stack the papers and staple them together along the left side to create a tree book. Together, identify the trees in your book and label each page with the appropriate tree name. If you like, look through a guide to the trees in your area to learn more.

Babies

While older playmates do this activity, you can use a tree to delight babies' senses. Rub babies' palms gently on bark and leaves to let them enjoy the different textures. Then lay the babies on a blanket under the tree to watch the leaves fluttering in the wind.

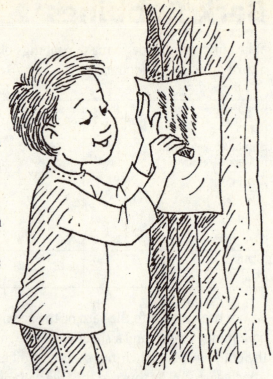

Toddlers

Toddlers may need assistance when making their rubbings, since they're still developing their ability to hold and manipulate objects such as crayons. Rubbing a tree with a rough surface may make it that much more challenging. Guide their hands to help them gently move their crayon up and down on the paper. They may only want to fill a small portion of the paper with the rubbing. Back inside, they can add a leaf rubbing, too. Set a leaf on the table, lay their paper over it, and tape it in place. They'll enjoy seeing the leaf outline appear as they rub the crayon on the paper over the leaf!

Preschoolers

Preschoolers' vocabulary is growing incredibly, especially with descriptive words. When inside, encourage them to describe their tree to you. Record the descriptions on their paper.

School-Age Children

Back inside, encourage school-age children to write a story or a poem on their papers about the many wonderful things trees provide, like shade, fruit, nuts, shelters for animals, and more.

Did You Know?
Each year, a mature, leafy tree produces as much oxygen as forty people inhale.

Sticking to Our ABCs

Use alphabet magnets to reinforce letter learning.

What You'll Need	All Ages	Babies	Toddlers	Preschoolers	School-Age Children
Metal baking sheets (or pans)	✋				
Alphabet magnets	✋				

Give each child a metal baking sheet, then spread out a set of alphabet magnets within reach of all children. No matter what their ages, the children will have fun moving, sorting, and arranging the letters.

Babies

It's never too early to introduce letters to a baby. If the baby is six months or older, place him in a highchair and let him have fun pushing the letters around a baking sheet. He'll enjoy pulling each letter off and putting it back on the sheet. For babies younger than six months, arrange the letters to spell their names on the sheet. Say each letter out loud as you place it on the sheet. Even though a baby won't recognize his name, the contrast of the colored letters against the shiny metal will attract his attention.

Toddlers

Toddlers will use this activity to practice their sorting and arranging skills more than their letter recognition. Toddlers may work hard to arrange the letters on their baking sheet, only to take them off and create a new arrangement on the table. Before they create a new arrangement, point to and name each letter for them.

Preschoolers

At this age, preschoolers may be discovering that letters come together to form words, including their own names. They may even make up words with the magnets and ask you what they spell. Play along and sound out their creations as best you can. This exercise is a wonderful way to build the foundation for reading.

School-Age Children

School-age children can read and spell, so give them a special challenge with the alphabet magnets. Help them create a long word at the top of their baking sheet, like *family* or *holiday*. Then ask them how many other words they can create by using just those letters.

Host Tip

If you don't have alphabet magnets, older children can create a homemade set. Cut out large letters from magazines, then glue the letters to small square pieces of cardboard cut out from a cereal box. Finally, stick a magnetic strip to the back of each piece.

Opposite Hunt

Room by room, playmates can explore opposites.

What You'll Need	All Ages	Babies	Toddlers	Preschoolers	School-Age Children
Notebook and pencil					✋

As a group, take a tour of your home and seek out opposites. Turn lights on and off. Fill a bucket with toys, then empty it. Go up a step, then down one. Make a happy face, then a sad one. Hold a piece of ice, then touch warm water. Hug a soft teddy bear, then touch the hard floor. Explain to the group that these objects, actions, and feelings are opposites.

Babies

Babies will love taking this tour with their playmates. Babies at least six months old can flick the light switch on and off, or take part in emptying the toy bins and filling them back up. Be sure to emphasize the opposite words as the baby does the actions: "The light is *on*. The light is *off*." This is an important time for babies to build vocabulary and link words to objects and effects. Younger babies will enjoy playing this simple opposites game: Wave and say, "Goodbye" as you walk away, then quickly return and wave and say, "Hello." They'll love the repetition and may want you to do it again and again.

Toddlers

During the tour, don't be surprised if toddlers become particularly enthralled with one activity (for example, turning on and off the lights). In addition to learning about opposites, they're learning about cause and effect, thinking, "I flip this switch, and a light goes on. I flip it again, and then it goes off," or, "I turn a knob, and the water turns on. I turn it again, and the water turns off." This activity helps them learn how their actions create results.

Preschoolers

Preschoolers can likely name the opposites of things they discover during the tour. To encourage them, say, "We are going up the step. What is the opposite of up?" or, "This water is cold. What's the opposite of cold?" Chances are, you will be surprised by all the opposites they know.

School-Age Children

School-age children can keep track of all the opposites the group discovers on the tour. Give them a notebook and a pencil, and have them write each pair of opposites ("up/down" or "on/off") as you come across them. Or they can go ahead of younger playmates and identify opposites in the next room. When others arrive, they may say, "I found five opposites in here. Can you find them?" Encourage them to give hints when necessary.

Host Tip

This activity can be a fun, clever way to remind children of manners or tidiness. For example, you may say, "This living room needs to be the opposite of messy!"

All About Us

Children will learn about themselves and one another with this fun activity!

What You'll Need	All Ages	Babies	Toddlers	Preschoolers	School-Age Children
Light-colored construction paper	✋				
Markers	✋				
Crayons and stickers	✋				
Photo					✋
Paper clips	✋				
Yarn	✋				
Tape	✋				
Tape measure					✋
Bathroom scale					✋

For each child, write the following list down the left side of a sheet of light-colored construction paper. School-age children can help with this task.

Name	Eye color
Birthday	Favorite color
Height	Favorite food
Weight	Favorite book
Hair color	Hobbies

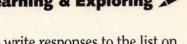

See below for ways to help children write responses to the list on their sheets. Then let them decorate their sheets with crayons or stickers. When the sheets are finished, use paper clips to secure them to a five-foot piece of yarn to make a banner. Use tape to prominently display the banner in your play area.

Babies

Have other children help you come up with a baby's responses. For example, they may suggest that eating or napping are hobbies. To determine the baby's favorite color, they can hold up toys in different colors and see which one gets the best reaction.

Toddlers

Toddlers may need help expressing their responses, which a helper can then write down. For example, when determining a favorite color, a helper may say, "Do you like red? Our couch is red. Or do you like blue? Your shirt is blue." You can also determine a favorite book by pointing to a few books they are familiar with and letting them decide on a favorite.

Preschoolers

Help preschoolers by recording their responses on their sheets. If they are learning to write, challenge them to write their name in the appropriate spot. For extra help, print their names on another sheet of paper and have them copy the letters on their sheets. When they are done, encourage them to draw a picture of themselves on the sheet. They can draw themselves doing one of their hobbies or enjoying one of their favorite things.

School-Age Children

At the beginning of the activity, school-age children can help measure and weigh the younger playmates. For a fun exercise, have them estimate the height and weight of each playmate before taking the measurements. After they fill in their own responses, have them glue a current photo of themselves onto the paper. Ask them to find a photo that emphasizes something from the list, such as brown eyes.

Host Tip

When you're done displaying the banner, be sure to store it in a safe place, or let the children take their sheets home. They will make great keepsakes for years to come, and children may enjoy looking at them as they grow.

Weather Watch

Track the local weather with these simple weather boards.

What You'll Need	All Ages	Babies	Toddlers	Preschoolers	School-Age Children
Index cards			🖐	🖐	🖐
Crayons			🖐	🖐	🖐
Poster board			🖐	🖐	🖐
Markers			🖐	🖐	🖐
Velcro			🖐	🖐	🖐
Tape			🖐	🖐	🖐
Weather thermometer				🖐	
Weather resources, such as newspapers or almanacs					🖐

As a group, discuss the weather conditions you experience in your area throughout the year (sunny, cloudy, windy, rainy, snowy, and so on). Have preschoolers and school-age children draw a picture on an index card for each of these weather conditions. They can then create their own weatherboards using large sheets of poster board. Write "Today's Weather" at the top, cut sticky-backed Velcro strips, and affix a loop half to the back of each card. Affix two or three (or more) hook halves to the construction paper. Do one set for each child to bring home. When you're done, have the kids look out a window or go outside to identify the current weather. Have them stick the appropriate card(s) to their boards. Tell the kids to keep these weather cards by a window, and each morning to display the cards that describe that day's weather. Below are some additional ways children can enjoy the weather boards as a group and at home.

Babies

While older children observe the weather, use the opportunity to teach a baby words that describe the weather. For example, say, "Look at the leaves blowing around on the ground. That means it's *windy*." If you like, further illustrate the weather by gently blowing on the baby's face to imitate wind. Take the baby to the window (or outside if properly dressed) to experience the weather as you describe it.

Toddlers

In addition to seeing the weather through a window, toddlers can feel the weather. For example, open a window or door and have them reach a hand outside. Ask, "How does that feel? Cold? Wet? Windy?" The tactile exercise will help toddlers connect words with their meanings.

Preschoolers

Preschoolers love to make their own decisions, so after determining the day's weather, have them decide what type of clothing they should wear. Should they wear a hat and scarf or sandals and shorts? Preschoolers may also want to know the temperature before choosing clothing, so display a thermometer outside a window. Use simple terms to explain how to read it. If it's a mercury thermometer, say, "The shorter the red line is, the colder it is outside. And the longer the red line is, the warmer it is."

School-Age Children

Challenge school-age children to forecast the next day's weather. They can continue these predictions once at home and may choose to watch a weather segment on the evening news; read the weather section in the daily paper; visit a weather website (with adult supervision); or read a book about weather predictions, like *The Old Farmer's Almanac for Kids*. They can then see whether their predictions are right!

Number Matchup

All kids will enjoy playing with these homemade number cards.

What You'll Need	All Ages	Babies	Toddlers	Preschoolers	School-Age Children
20 index cards	🖐				
Crayons	🖐				
Small stickers	🖐				

Help children create two sets of ten index cards. On one set, number the cards 1 through 10 (one number per card). On the other set, place one sticker on the first card, two stickers on the second card, three stickers on the third card, and so on until you place ten stickers on the tenth card. Once they're finished, children can play the following age-appropriate games with the cards.

Babies

Teach other children to recite the following rhyme to the baby. Each time they say a number, they can hold up both its numeral and sticker cards. The baby will enjoy watching the cards and listening to the rhyme.

> *One, two—we love you.*
> *Three, four—we'll teach you more.*
> *Five, six—[baby's name] we pick.*
> *Seven, eight—arms out straight.*
> *Nine, ten—we hug again!*

Toddlers

Help toddlers begin to recognize numbers using the cards. Place a sticker card in front of them and ask, "How many stickers do you see here?" Count out loud together as you point to each sticker. Say, "One, two—I see two stickers." Then show them the corresponding numeral card and say, "This is the number 2."

Preschoolers

Preschoolers can play a memory game with the cards. Show them how to shuffle the two sets of cards  together, then lay them face-down in five rows. Have them turn over one card, then turn over another card. If they match a sticker card to its corresponding numeral card, they keep both. If they don't match, turn them back over. See how many turns it takes to match all the pairs, then challenge preschoolers to play again and try to lower that number.

School-Age Children

Here's a fun, challenging math game for school-age children: Have them randomly pick a sticker card. Tell them that number is the "answer" to a math problem—one they must create with the numeral cards! For instance, if they drew the card with 7 stickers, they could then pick up the 3 and 4 numeral cards because 3 plus 4 equals 7. Or they could pick up the 10 and 3 numeral cards because 10 minus 3 is 7.

Window Painting

Let children practice writing in an unusual way—by painting on a window!

What You'll Need	All Ages	Babies	Toddlers	Preschoolers	School-Age Children
Newspaper, tape, and large sheet	🖐				
Old T-shirts or smocks	🖐				
Window paint (1 part powdered tempera paint and 1 part clear liquid dishwasher detergent)	🖐				
Shallow bowls	🖐				
Paintbrushes	🖐				

Choose a large glass window or door all kids can easily reach. The paint will wash off glass, but tape newspaper to the wall below the glass and spread a large sheet on the floor. Have children put on old T-shirts or smocks to protect their clothes as well. Then mix different-colored batches of window paint and pour the paint into shallow bowls. Give kids each a paintbrush and a bowl, assign them a section of glass, and let them start painting!

Babies

Babies six months or older can hold small paintbrushes and write a letter or draw a line with your help. If you like, let babies move the paintbrush themselves to make their own works of art! If the baby is younger, make sure all playmates use brightly colored paint to catch a baby's interest.

Toddlers

Toddlers will love to make their mark on the glass! Show them how to dip the paintbrush in the paint, then brush it lightly on the glass. Assist by helping each to write the first letter of their names on the window. Mention the shapes and lines found in that letter and say them as you paint together. For example, say, "*B* is for Brooke. Let's draw a straight line and then two half circles to make a *B*."

Preschoolers

If possible, assign preschoolers to a window or door with a lattice. (Some windows have the lattice part encased in the window, but for those that have wooden exposed lattice, it will be best to protect that area with some painters' tape.) Challenge them to spell their name or another simple word one letter per pane. If you don't have a lattice, draw some on the glass for them to use. If necessary, spell words for them letter by letter as they write.

School-Age Children

Have school-age children practice writing in different sizes. For example, they can write very small letters with a small paintbrush and very large letters with a large paintbrush. If they are learning how to write in cursive, this activity is a fun, artistic way to practice!

What Floats?

In this activity, children will discover which items float and which ones sink.

What You'll Need	All Ages	Babies	Toddlers	Preschoolers	School-Age Children
Immersible objects, including a small ball, rock, bottle cap, apple or orange, Ping-Pong ball, cotton ball, metal fork, wooden block, bath toys, marbles, and so on	🖑				
Large clear bowl	🖑				
Small bowl		🖑			
Clear plastic bottle		🖑			

To begin, gather a variety of small immersible objects from around the house. Then fill a large clear bowl with water and have children gather around it. Ask them whether they think each item will float or sink. Take turns testing each item by dropping it into the bowl.

Babies

While babies watch older children discover which objects sink or float, they can experiment with water, too. Babies six months or older can sit in a highchair, with a small bowl of water in front of them. Place a Ping-Pong ball (or other floatable ball) in the water, and encourage the baby to reach for it. For younger babies, fill a clear plastic bottle with water and drop in a marble.

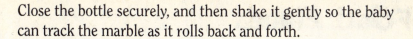

Close the bottle securely, and then shake it gently so the baby can track the marble as it rolls back and forth.

Toddlers

Show toddlers what *floating* means to help them understand the purpose of the activity. First put a light object, like a Ping-Pong ball, in the bowl. Then say, "See the ball on top of the water? It's floating." Then remove the light item and drop a heavy object, like a rock, into the water. Say, "See the rock on the bottom of the bowl? It's *not* floating." As you continue with the activity, make sure each toddler gets plenty of opportunities to drop items into the water to help hold their interest.

Preschoolers and School-Age Children

Discuss with preschoolers and school-age children why certain items float and others sink. What do they think the reason is? Let them discover that even if items weigh the same, they may not float or sink the same. For example, have them test this idea with a wooden block and a steel fork. What do they think will happen? Are their predictions correct?

Host Tip

To introduce the concepts of sinking and floating, read *Who Sank the Boat?* by Pamela Allen with your children.

Did You Know?
An object will float if it weighs as much as the water it displaces. The heavier it is, the more water it needs to displace in order to float.

Food Plates

Make colorful food plates to teach kids about healthy eating.

What You'll Need	All Ages	Babies	Toddlers	Preschoolers	School-Age Children
Large sheets of orange, green, red, purple, blue, and yellow construction paper	👋				
Markers	👋				
Grocery flyers and magazines	👋				
Child-safe scissors	👋				
Glue sticks	👋				

Cut large triangles out of orange, green, red, and purple construction paper, one of each color for each child. Make the green triangles bigger than the others. If you like, round one side of each triangle so you do not end up with square plates! Then cut large circles out of blue construction paper, one circle per child. Label the pieces with the following food group names, coordinating the labels with the colors used in the United States Department of Agriculture (USDA) myplate.gov food guidance system:

- Grains (orange)
- Vegetables (green)
- Fruits (red)
- Protein (purple)
- Dairy (blue)

Help the children assemble their plates on the yellow construction paper to look like the diagram below. Once the plates are ready, take a few minutes to discuss each food group with the children. For example, say, "The dairy group not only includes the milk we drink but also foods made from milk, like yogurt and cheese." Together, look through grocery flyers and magazines for pictures of foods, helping them determine which items belong in which groups. Finally, have them cut out the images and glue each onto the appropriate color.

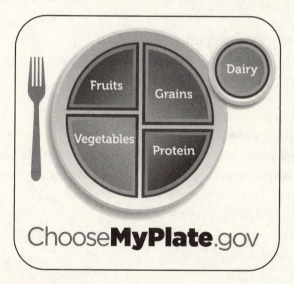

Babies and Toddlers

Team up with babies and toddlers for this activity, which can be a great vocabulary builder. As you find and cut out images, hold up each one and say what it is and what food group it belongs to. For example, you can show them a picture of an apple and say, "This is an apple. It's a fruit." Then spread the glue on the back of the image and let a toddler press it onto the correct color on her plate.

Preschoolers

Challenge preschoolers to find images to fill certain food groups. For example, say, "We need another picture for our vegetable group. Can you find a vegetable?" Or have them find specific images that make up a balanced diet, such as dark green or orange vegetables.

School-Age Children

As a special assignment, have school-age children cut out only foods they have never eaten before.

Host Tip

If the children like, they can put small star stickers next to foods they've tried at least once. This exercise may encourage them to earn more stars by trying the foods they've been avoiding!

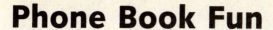

Phone Book Fun

Let children have some fun with an old phone book before recycling it.

What You'll Need	All Ages	Babies	Toddlers	Preschoolers	School-Age Children
Old phone book	✋				
Crayons			✋		
Highlighter				✋	
Watch or timer					✋

Divide an old phone book into sections, one for each child, by opening the book flat and ripping along the spine. Give a section to each child, and let them have fun exploring the pages in different ways.

Babies

Babies six months or older can crumple a page or two in their fists, enjoying the paper's texture and the crinkling sound it makes. Crumple the pages for younger babies yourself, or ask an older playmate to do it. You may also want to gently fan a baby with a few pages. She'll enjoy the cool breeze.

Toddlers

Toddlers will love ripping out the phone book pages. When each has torn out some pages, help them find the first letter of their name on them. Circle each find with a crayon and say something like, "There's a *B*. *B* is for Brooke. That's you! Can you find another *B*?"

Preschoolers

You can challenge preschoolers by calling out a random number for them to find in the phone book. For example, ask them to find the number 4, then have them use a highlighter to mark all the 4s they can find on one page. This phone book activity is the perfect time to have them recite their own phone numbers and even practice dialing it.

School-Age Children

School-age children can practice alphabetization skills with their phone book section. Point out the words or names at the top of each page, and explain that they are the first and last entries on that page. Then have them rip out a number of pages, mix them up, and put them back into alphabetical order. If you like, time them, then challenge them to mix up the pages again and try to beat their time.

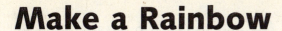

Make a Rainbow

Dazzle children by using simple science to create an indoor rainbow!

What You'll Need	All Ages	Babies	Toddlers	Preschoolers	School-Age Children
Compact mirror	🖐				
Empty clear glass jar	🖐				
Pitcher of water	🖐				
Flashlight	🖐				
Crayons, markers, and construction paper			🖐	🖐	🖐

Gather a compact mirror, clear glass jar, pitcher of water, and flashlight, and head to a darkened room with the group. (A room with light-colored walls will let kids see rainbows the best.) Place the compact mirror, tilted slightly upward, into the jar. A preschooler can help pour water into the jar, then have a school-age child shine a flashlight through the water and onto the mirror. A rainbow will appear on the wall opposite the mirror. If one doesn't, change the angle of the flashlight or mirror. Children can enjoy the rainbow in the following age-appropriate ways:

Babies

Hold a baby close to the rainbow so he can see the array of colors. (That is, if being in a dark room doesn't just lull him to sleep!)

Toddlers

Encourage toddlers to touch the rainbow. Depending on where it is, they may need to reach high and jump, or crouch low.

Preschoolers

Ask preschoolers to identify the shape of the rainbow and name the colors they see in it.

School-age children

Challenge school-age children to change the angle of the mirror or shine the flashlight at a different angle to make rainbows in other locations around the room.

Host Tips
- Discuss the "magic" behind making a rainbow: Light is made up of all the colors. When water mixes with light, it acts as a prism, which means it breaks the light into seven main colors: red, orange, yellow, green, blue, indigo, and violet.
- Discuss how the indoor rainbow is similar to and different from the rainbow they see in the sky after it rains.
- Follow up by having children draw their own rainbows with crayons or markers.

Name Plates

What's in a name? Children can find out during this fun activity.

What You'll Need	All Ages	Babies	Toddlers	Preschoolers	School-Age Children
Child-safe scissors	✋				
Construction paper	✋				
Baby name book	✋				
Crayons and stickers	✋				
Clear contact paper	✋				

Help children cut out three-inch-by-nine-inch rectangles from construction paper. With the help of a baby-name book, like one of the many by Bruce Lansky (Meadowbrook Press), write the meaning of each child's name along the bottom of a rectangle, then write the child's name above the meaning in larger letters. (Older children may do this step themselves or with some help.) Toddlers, preschoolers, and school-age children can then decorate their nameplates and the baby's with crayons and stickers.

When each nameplate is done, cover both sides with clear contact paper and trim the excess. Families can use the nameplates to label shelf space or toy boxes, assign seats at the dining table, and more!

Babies

A baby's name is one of the first words he'll recognize and understand. Introduce him to the written form of his name by tracing his finger over the letters on his nameplate. Also encourage older kids to play a game of peekaboo so the baby can hear his name. For example, his playmates can say, "Where's [baby's name]?" while covering their eyes with his nameplate. Then they can uncover their eyes quickly while saying, "There's [baby's name]!" He'll love the interaction.

Toddlers

This activity is a great way to introduce toddlers to writing. Help toddlers write their names on their nameplates. Show them how to hold a crayon between a thumb and index finger, then guide their hands with your own as you write the names. Make sure to identify each letter as you write it.

Preschoolers

Preschoolers may need help spelling their names. If they do, write the names on scraps of construction paper so they can use them as guides. When they are ready to decorate the nameplates, encourage them to draw objects that begin with each letter of their name. For example, if a preschooler's name is Jack, ask him to draw a jet, apple, cat, and key.

School-Age Children

If you like, put school-age children in charge of finding all the names in the baby-name book. Have them read the meanings to you, or they can write them on the nameplates themselves. Encourage them to share with their playmates whatever they discover about their names.

Head, Shoulders, Knees, and Toes

Here's a fun, well-known song that teaches kids about their bodies.

What You'll Need	All Ages	Babies	Toddlers	Preschoolers	School-Age Children
Blanket		🖐			

Use the following song to teach kids about the different parts of their bodies.

> *Head, shoulders, knees, and toes,*
> *knees and toes.*
> *Head, shoulders, knees, and toes,*
> *knees and toes.*
> *Eyes and ears*
> *and mouth and nose.*
> *Head, shoulders, knees, and toes,*
> *knees and toes.*

Each time a body part is mentioned, encourage older children to touch or point to the corresponding part. Below you'll find other age-appropriate ways to enjoy the song.

Babies

Help babies learn about their bodies through infant massage. This technique benefits both baby and parent as it gives special time for bonding, promotes relaxation, and may improve a baby's sleep. Lay a baby on a blanket and sing the song, using your fingertips to gently rub the baby's scalp and massage shoulders, knees, and toes.

Toddlers

At about thirteen months old, toddlers may be able to identify one body part. At about eighteen months old, they may identify up to six body parts. Before singing, help them identify their head, shoulders, knees, and toes. For example, ask, "Where is your head? It's right here!" (Point to head.) "Where are your toes? That's right. There they are!" (Point to toes.)

Preschoolers

Most preschoolers can identify the major parts of their bodies. After singing "Head, Shoulders, Knees, and Toes" a few times, make it fun by speeding up or by changing a body part to touch. For instance, sing, "Head, shoulders, knees, and elbows."

School-Age Children

School-age children are ready to learn about the internal parts of their bodies. Discuss the many systems in their body, including cardiovascular, respiratory, nervous, and digestive, and name some of the main organs in each system. Then sing

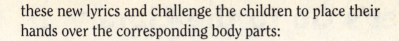

these new lyrics and challenge the children to place their hands over the corresponding body parts:

Brain, stomach, heart and lungs,
heart and lungs.
Brain, stomach, heart and lungs,
heart and lungs.
Throat and tongue—
all inside.
Brain, stomach, heart and lungs,
heart and lungs.

Did You Know?
There are 206 bones in the human body, and most of them are in the hands and feet.

Let's Go to the Library

There's nothing better than visiting the local library together!

What You'll Need	All Ages	Babies	Toddlers	Preschoolers	School-Age Children
A love of books!	✋				

Whether it's your first trip to the library as a group or your hundredth, here are some ways to make it a fun, educational experience.

Babies

When visiting the library, ask a librarian for the staff's recommendations for babies. You'll discover some wonderful titles! It's important to read to babies every day. Hearing the stories will help language development, and snuggling together makes reading time special. A baby six months or older can help choose a book to check out. Hold up two brightly colored books and see which one the baby moves toward.

Toddlers

Toddlerhood is a busy, important time. Toddlers will greatly benefit from books that feature other kids and how they deal with real issues, such as using the potty or sleeping in a big bed. Their vocabulary is also growing tremendously and can be reinforced through reading together. Be sure to check out books that discuss the events and issues in their life, plus let them choose a few board books about objects or characters they are currently into, like trains or ducks.

Preschoolers

Before visiting the library, ask the preschoolers what they want to learn more about. For example, if dinosaurs fascinate one of them, encourage them to look for books about dinosaurs. To help them further understand how the library can be a learning resource, help them ask a librarian for book suggestions on their favorite topics.

School-Age Children

School-age children can find books on their own. Show them how to use the library's electronic catalog to locate books by call number, then show them how to find the number by reading the labels on the bookcases and shelves. After finding their own books, they can help younger playmates find books that interest them.

Host Tip

Here are some other things to keep in mind for your next trip to the library:

- Your library may offer fun activities for all ages, from story hours to arts-and-crafts activities to holiday celebrations. Make sure to grab a calendar of events during your visit.
- Letting school-age children have their own library card will make them feel responsible and independent.

Money! Money! Money!

It is never too early to discuss money with children. A great way to get started is to have them create their own banks.

What You'll Need	All Ages	Babies	Toddlers	Preschoolers	School-Age Children
Coins	✋				
Empty plastic bottles		✋			✋
Empty milk cartons			✋	✋	
Construction paper			✋	✋	
Glue			✋	✋	
Scissors			✋	✋	
Stickers			✋		
Markers				✋	✋
Masking tape					✋

Babies

Let babies watch as you or an older child drops coins into an empty plastic bottle. Name each coin (quarter, dime, nickel, and penny) as you do so. Once the bottle is securely closed, allow the baby to shake it and see the coins move about.

Toddlers

Help toddlers make their own banks. For each child, cover an empty milk carton with construction paper, cut a slit for the coins, and let them decorate their banks with stickers. When they are done, they'll have fun dropping coins into the bank. Teach them how to open the carton to release the coins and start all over again. *Note*: Close parental supervision is required because coins pose a choking risk.

Preschoolers

Preschoolers can also make banks from milk cartons. For each child, cover the carton with construction paper, cut a slit, and let them decorate the bank any way they choose. Or if they want to make their bank into a fire truck, use red construction paper and have them draw wheels, windows, and a ladder with a black marker. To make a dog, use brown construction paper and have them draw faces on it. You could even attach a long strip of brown construction paper as a tail. Before having them add coins to their banks, have them sort the coins by value.

School-Age Children

Are the school-age children earning money for chores around the house? (See "Helping Hands" on page 240 for ideas about age-appropriate chores.) If so, experts recommend teaching children how to deal with money responsibly. Provide each child with three bottles: Label one for spending, one for saving, and one for charity. They can cover their bottles with masking tape and then color them with markers. At the end of each month, they can go shopping with their spending money and decide where to send their donations.

Host Tip

Go to a local bank and get some coin wraps. Older children may enjoy sorting loose change, plus they'll see how quickly coins can add up!

A Shapely Mural

Playmates can use all sorts of cut-out shapes to make a mural.

What You'll Need	All Ages	Babies	Toddlers	Preschoolers	School-Age Children
Pencil	✋				
Child-safe scissors	✋				
Construction paper in various colors	✋				
Tape	✋				
Large sheet of paper (or poster board)	✋				
Glue sticks			✋	✋	✋

Begin by helping the children draw and cut out various geometric shapes from different-colored construction paper. Then tape a sheet of paper (or poster board) to the wall or lay it on a table where everyone can reach it. Have kids arrange the cut-out shapes into objects, scenes, or designs, then have them glue the shapes onto the paper. When finished, this mural will make a creative backdrop in a playroom or other prominent place.

Babies

While older playmates work on the mural, hold up some of the cut-out shapes and describe them to the baby. For example, say, "This is a square, and this is a triangle." Put the shapes on a highchair tray and guide the baby's finger around them.

Babies will also enjoy watching the mural come together with its bright, contrasting colors and shapes.

Toddlers

Help toddlers identify the various shapes, and encourage them to add them to the mural. For example, ask, "Can you find a circle and help me glue it onto the mural?" Cover the shape with glue and let them decide where to place it on the mural. You may also want to challenge toddlers to find cutouts by shape as well as color: "Can you find a blue triangle?"

Preschoolers

Challenge preschoolers to create a scene with the shapes. For example, they can use three circles to make a snowman next to a square house with a triangle roof. They may want to arrange the shapes on the floor or table first, then glue them onto the mural.

School-Age Children

Encourage school-age children to use the shapes to re-create a favorite memory, like sledding or drinking hot cocoa with friends. For instance, they could use a rectangle to make a sled or a square with an oval on top to create a mug of hot chocolate. Have them write a description of the memory next to their artwork.

Chapter 7

Team Friends

I remember the first time my husband and I witnessed our kids getting along and helping each other out. This miracle may be one of our proudest moments as parents!

—Heather

Somewhere in the midst of the hustle and bustle of life, children and their parents or guardians learn to work together and truly bond. That's what this chapter focuses on. Whether these activities encourage kids to cooperate with household chores or celebrate each other's birthdays, they'll teach children what it means to be a team. Children will discover how they can be an important part of their family or playgroup, but they'll also discover how wonderful friendship can be.

Me and My Friends Scrapbook

Children will love to a make scrapbook that celebrates them!

What You'll Need	All Ages	Babies	Toddlers	Preschoolers	School-Age Children
Family photos (or copies)	🖐				
Construction paper	🖐				
Glue sticks	🖐				
Markers			🖐	🖐	🖐
Stickers			🖐	🖐	🖐
Stapler	🖐				
Clear contact paper		🖐			

Before doing this activity, ask playmates to bring photos of themselves to the get-together. They'll want to make sure they have at least three to four pictures each, and maybe a few family images as well. Each child will use photos of himself for his own scrapbook page. If you want to preserve the originals, make copies. When it's time for the activity, give each child several sheets of construction paper. Help the children glue their photos onto the front and back of each page. If they like, they can add a caption under each photo and decorate the pages with markers and stickers. After the children finish their pages, stack them, then staple them together along the left side to create a book for each child.

Babies

Hold the baby in your lap as you create scrapbook pages. While you glue photos onto the paper, tell the baby about what's going on in each photo. For babies older than six months, choose a few additional photos of her family, glue them onto a separate sheet of paper, then cover the sheet with clear contact paper. Give the sheet to the baby so she can see the images of her loved ones close up.

Toddlers

You can help toddlers make their pages by dabbing glue on the backs of the photos and letting them press the photos into place on the paper. Then point to each photo and ask a question such as, "Who is that?" Write their responses near the photos, even if it's simply, "Me!"

Preschoolers

Preschoolers will enjoy showcasing their photos. Let them arrange and glue them onto the pages as they like. They can add their own special touches to the pages with stickers and markers. Ask them to give you a caption to include near each photo.

School-Age Children

In addition to designing their own scrapbook pages, school-age children may enjoy creating a special cover page for the book that includes a title. Add the cover to the top of the stack before you staple the pages together.

Host Tip
This activity is perfect after an outing with the group. It's a great way for kids to record the fun they had together. If you have a digital camera and a printer, take lots of pictures of the kids playing together during an outing or event, print them when you get home (on regular paper is fine), and let the children assemble their keepsake albums!

Family Trees

Create family trees made of real branches and homemade leaves.

What You'll Need	All Ages	Babies	Toddlers	Preschoolers	School-Age Children
12-inch branch	✋				
Modeling clay	✋				
Large plastic cup	✋				
Pencils	✋				
Cardstock	✋				
Child-safe scissors	✋				
Green construction paper	✋				
Ink pad	✋				
Crayons	✋				
Stickers	✋				
Paper clips	✋				
Wet wipes	✋				

In your yard or neighborhood, each playmate should find a twelve-inch branch with several small twigs. Place modeling clay at the bottom of large plastic cups. Stick the branches upright in the cups, using the modeling clay to secure them in place. Next, draw a leaf pattern that's six inches long on cardstock, then cut it out. Preschoolers and school-age children can trace the pattern on green construction paper, then cut out the shape to create leaves for themselves and for their younger playmates. Each child will need enough leaves for each member of their family (don't forget pets!). Children can then write names (with help, for the younger ones) on the back of their leaves and decorate the other side with crayons or stickers. Use paper clips to attach each leaf to a twig on the branch to create individual family trees.

Babies

A baby can help create his own leaf. Gently press his thumb onto an ink pad and then onto the leaf several times to create a fun design or even to write his name with thumbprints. Have wet wipes nearby to clean his hand when you're done. While designing his leaf, sing this song to the tune of "I'm a Little Teapot":

> *I'm a little baby, special and small.*
> *Here is my family; I love them all.*
> *When we add the branches to this tree,*
> *See the names of my family.*

Before attaching the baby's leaf to the branch, let him admire the artwork he helped create!

Toddlers

Write the toddlers' names in big bubble letters on the back of their leaves. If any name is too long to fit, write initials instead. Say each letter as you write it. Let the toddlers use crayons to color in the bubble letters.

Preschoolers

After the preschoolers have decorated one side of their leaves, help them write their name and the names of other family members on the other side. Have them hold a crayon, then put your hand over theirs. Print each name on the leaf while guiding their hands, so they can practice writing and strengthen their hand movements. Make sure to say each letter as you write it. If a preschooler knows how to write their name, challenge them to write it with bubble letters.

School-Age Children
School children can create leaves for parents, grandparents, aunts, uncles, and cousins too.

Host Tip
If you like, playmates can add a decorative touch to their completed family trees: Think up a title for their trees, such as "The Smith Family" or "Our Family Tree." Cut a piece of brightly colored fabric to cover the large plastic cup, and write the title on it with fabric markers. When you're done, glue the fabric around the plastic cup.

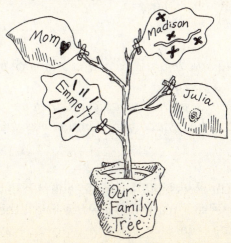

Questions in the Jar

Make mealtime a special time by playing this fun question game.

What You'll Need	All Ages	Babies	Toddlers	Preschoolers	School-Age Children
Glass jar or plastic container					
Paper	🖐				
Pen	🖐				

Find a clean, empty glass jar or plastic container to place on the center of your dining room table. On separate slips of paper, write questions about the children's thoughts, interests, and dreams. Here are some examples:

- *What is the best thing about being the age you are?*
- *What would be a perfect day for you?*
- *Who is your favorite friend? Why?*
- *If you could have any animal as a pet, which would you choose?*
- *If you could take a family vacation anyplace in the world, where would you go?*
- *If you had three wishes, what would they be?*
- *Do you know how much your family loves you? How can you tell?*

When done writing questions, put the slips in the jar. At mealtime or snack time, have children take turns picking slips from the jar and answering the questions. In no time, there will be a lively, pleasant conversation at the dinner table!

Babies

Although babies can't converse verbally, they'll enjoy hearing loved ones' voices and seeing their faces. When it's a baby's turn to draw a slip, you can either answer the question for her or ask the other children what they think the baby's answer would be.

Toddlers

Toddlers will need some help when it's their turn. Read the question for them, then elicit an answer by asking yes-or-no questions about the topic, such as, "Do you like puppies? Would you like one as a pet? Do you like kitties, too?" Or instead of asking toddlers the question from the jar, consider asking them simpler questions, such as, "Was it cold out today?" "Did you play with a friend today?" or, "Did any books you read today have animals in them?" Either way, they'll enjoy demonstrating their growing vocabulary and cognitive skills.

Preschoolers and School-Age Children

After preschoolers and school-age children have replied to their respective questions on the slips, ask them additional questions to expand their answers. For example, if a school-age child answers, "Alaska," to the question about an ideal vacation spot, you may say, "What do you think Alaska would be like if you went there on a family vacation?"

Host Tip

Mealtime is not only a great chance for children to practice the art of conversation, but it's also a great chance for them to practice good manners. Children can be silly and loud when they get talking. Help promote good listening skills by reminding children to take turns talking and to use proper voice levels at the dinner table. Also encourage children to use polite words like *please* and *thank you*. The more they use these words, the more of a habit it will become. Teach children— including babies—the American Sign Language (ASL) signs for common words used at mealtime. (See page 245 for more signs.) For example:

- *Thank you*: Raise your right hand—palm facing you, fingers together, and thumb pressed to the side of the hand—and touch the fingertips to your lips. Then bring your hand down and away from your mouth.
- *Please*: Make small circles on your chest with an open hand.

Start Your Day Right

What needs to happen each morning to get up and ready?
Create these visual guides and start off each day right!

What You'll Need	All Ages	Babies	Toddlers	Preschoolers	School-Age Children
Magazines or crayons			✋	✋	✋
Child-safe scissors			✋	✋	✋
Construction paper	✋				
Glue	✋				
Photos		✋			

Work with children to think up a list of tasks each child must
do each morning, like making the bed, brushing teeth and
hair, eating breakfast, and putting on shoes. Make sure the
tasks are age appropriate. Then have toddlers, preschoolers,
and school-age children find magazine images that depict
their important morning tasks, or you can help them draw the
images. With your help, each child can cut out and glue the
images onto a sheet of construction paper to make a guide.
Tell the children to post the guides in a spot at home where
they can see them every morning. They can use the guides to
get these tasks done quickly and while having fun!

Babies

While older playmates make their guides, show babies pictures
of people eating, playing, or getting dressed. Show them each

photo as you talk about it. Then glue the photos to a sheet of construction paper to hang in their kitchen.

Toddlers

Help toddlers find three pictures that depict their morning routines. Cut out each image, then ask them to tell you what's happening in it: "What is this boy doing? Is he brushing his teeth? Show me how you brush your teeth." Dab glue on the back of each cutout and let toddlers press them onto the construction paper. When finished, point to the images and explain how they make up their morning routine. For example, "When you wake up in the morning, first you brush your teeth, then you eat breakfast and get dressed."

Preschoolers

To strengthen preschoolers' sense of sequencing, have them glue their images onto the paper in the proper order. What do they do first? What do they do second? What do they do last? If necessary, here's your chance to try to change a routine! Offer suggestions, such as, "Do you think it may work better if you get dressed after breakfast, so if you spill something on your shirt you won't have to change again?"

School-Age Children

As school-age children prepare to leave for school each morning, their routines may be rushed. When making the guides, encourage them to create a timeline to accompany their images. For example, they can note the hour when they need to wake up to get things done. They may even want their guide to begin the evening before. For example, they can depict setting out the next day's clothes and note the time when they should do this task the previous night.

When my son started preschool, we created this guide. Instead of just telling him it was time to get dressed, I could point to the image on the guide and give him a visual cue as well. He liked running to check what task was next.

—Heather

Helping Hands

This is a wonderful activity to encourage teamwork among playmates and also one they can take home and use with their families.

What You'll Need	All Ages	Babies	Toddlers	Preschoolers	School-Age Children
Construction paper	🖐				
Crayons	🖐				
Child-safe scissors	🖐				
Envelopes	🖐				
Tape	🖐				

To begin this activity, have each child place a hand on a sheet of construction paper, then trace around the hand. With older children's help, cut out the tracings and use each one to create at least five more hand cutouts per child. Place each set of hand cutouts in a separate labeled envelope.

Explain to children that the cutouts are "helping hands," which represent times when the children have been helpful to someone. Every time a child does a helpful act, one of his or her hand cutouts should be taped to the wall, refrigerator door, or other highly visible place. Start awarding "helping hands" by recalling a helpful act each child did recently. For example, you may say to a school-age child, "Remember the time you helped a friend with her homework? That was very helpful." After acknowledging the helpful act, record it on one of his hand cutouts and tape it to the wall. Encourage the playmates to acknowledge one another's helpful acts and continue to add cutouts to the wall. By seeing all their "helping hands," the group will understand how much their contributions mean to their friends. Have each child make extra hands to bring home so they can continue this activity with their families.

Babies

Although a baby can't help in the same ways her older playmates can, she can make her friends feel loved and special by snuggling, cooing, smiling, or even listening intently. Be sure to point out baby's helpful contributions to her friends. For example, if a playmate seems out of sorts, you can say to him, "See the baby smiling at you? She wants you to be happy, too!" At home, a baby's hand cutouts will make great keepsakes as well as help chart her development.

Toddlers

At this age, toddlers are beginning to empathize and sympathize with others. If toddlers see a friend cry, they may try to help by offering a teddy bear, a hug, or just a caring glance. Help toddlers understand the connection between receiving a hand cutout and doing a helpful act. For example, say, "You made your friend feel better by giving her a hug." Also verbalize your own helpful actions. For example, "I'm giving your friend a hug because he's feeling sad."

Preschoolers

Most preschoolers like to exert their newfound independence. At this point, they can dress themselves, put on their shoes,

Team Friends

and even make their beds. Preschoolers are at the perfect age to assist their younger friends with these tasks. Encourage them to help a younger friend learn to pull on socks or take off their shoes.

School-Age Children
School-age children may be ready to help in more-involved ways. For example, you can suggest that they make a snack for the group or pick out a game. At home, they can help set the table, fold laundry, or feed the dog. Challenge them to come up with other ways they can help.

Host Tip
Encourage parents to continue to acknowledge their children's helpful acts with helpful hands at home and keep it up at play-groups too. This is a great way to reinforce good manners and the values of being a good friend!

Letters for Family

Work with children to write their own family letters to send to someone special.

What You'll Need	All Ages	Babies	Toddlers	Preschoolers	School-Age Children
Paper, pencil, envelope, and stamp	🖐				
Scale and tape measure		🖐			
Ink pad		🖐			
Wet wipes		🖐			
Stickers			🖐	🖐	
Crayons				🖐	

Gather around the kitchen table and tell the children they are each going to write a family letter. To get started, they can brainstorm about their accomplishments and news. Ask each child questions such as, "What makes you happy?" and, "What have you learned to do that makes you proud?" Write down their answers. The children can then create a letter to mail to someone they love.

Babies

Babies can't express themselves verbally, so let playmates help answer questions about baby's accomplishments. The recipient of the letter will surely want to know how much the baby has grown, so let older children help weigh and measure their friend with a scale and tape measure. Encourage older kids to hug and kiss the baby as they take his measurements. Have the baby "sign" the finished letter with a handprint. Press the palm side of his hand onto an ink pad, then press it onto the letter. Have wet wipes nearby for cleanup.

Toddlers

Make sure to ask toddlers open-ended questions as well as yes-or-no questions. For example, ask, "What did you do today?" and, "Do you want to tell your Grandma about your favorite toy?" This exercise will build vocabulary. You may also want to let toddlers decorate the backs of their envelopes with stickers.

Preschoolers

Preschoolers may enjoy talking at length about all their accomplishments. Challenge them to narrow their answers to just the most important ones. After the questions, they can contribute to the letter in many ways: They can decorate the borders of their finished letters with crayons and stickers, and they may be able to write their own name to sign it. If they like, they can draw portraits of family members to include with their letters. Finally, let them place the stamp on their envelope in the appropriate space.

School-Age Children

School-age children may enjoy writing the letters using the answers you recorded (with your help, if needed). Explain the basic parts of a formal letter: the date, the greeting, the main body, and a closing with everyone's names. Tell them where to write each part.

Show Me a Sign

Show children how to communicate without saying a word!

What You'll Need	All Ages	Babies	Toddlers	Preschoolers	School-Age Children
Hands!	✋				
ASL resource, such as a dictionary or website	✋				

Many parents use American Sign Language (ASL) to communicate with their children. See the chart on page 247 for signs to identify family members and feel free to consult an ASL resource to learn more. Repeat each sign several times as you say the corresponding word.

Babies

Babies can control their hand movements before they can speak, and they can recognize a sign well before they start using it on their own. These facts mean you can start using signs with a baby from birth. In addition to the signs on page 247, other important signs you may wish to teach baby include:

- *More*: Bring fingertips of both hands together and tap lightly.
- *Milk*: Open and close your right hand repeatedly as if milking a cow.
- *Eat*: Touch the fingertips and thumb of your right hand to your lips.
- *Drink*: Form a C shape with your right hand, then bring it up in a short arc to your mouth as if drinking from a glass.

Toddlers

Sign language will build toddlers' growing vocabulary. Sign often and encourage them to sign, too. For example, point to the baby and ask, "Who is this? Can you tell me with a sign?"

Preschoolers

Using sign language requires preschoolers to look at the person communicating with them, which may help them pay attention. Practice signing with preschoolers in everyday communication. For instance, you may ask, "Can you get a toy for your...?" and then sign *brother*. As preschoolers master making the signs, challenge them to come up with more signs to learn. For example, they may want to know how to sign their favorite activity or food. Find out how to make these signs together.

School-Age Children

In the signing community, each person makes a sign to represent his or her name. Encourage school-age children to create signs to represent their names. They may also enjoy learning the sign language alphabet. You can find the signs for each letter in your ASL resource. After they've learned the signs for the letters, challenge them to spell some words using the signs.

> *More* is one of the best signs for kids to learn! It can mean more food, more hugs, more throwing the ball; it can really help to keep a playdate going!
>
> —Lisa

Signs for Family Members & Friends	
Word	How to Make the Sign
Mommy	With an open right hand, touch your thumb to your chin and wiggle your fingers slightly.
Daddy	With an open right hand, touch your thumb to your forehead and wiggle your fingers slightly.
Friend	Interlock the index fingers twice.
Play	Make the Y sign with both hands and shake them.
Brother	Grasp the brim of an imaginary cap with your right thumb and fingers.
Sister	Tuck the fingers of your right hand, touch that thumb to your cheek, and sweep the thumb down the side of your face to your chin. Then bring both hands side by side in front of your chest, extending your index fingers straight out and tucking your other fingers.
Baby	Sway your arms together as if rocking a baby.

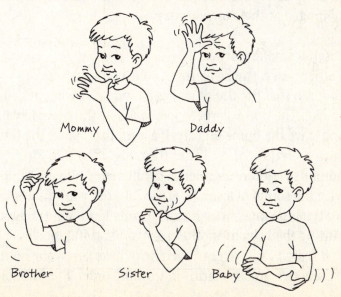

Mommy Daddy

Brother Sister Baby

Friend Fire Safety Plan

It's important to have a plan in case of fire in your home, and it's critical to teach it to children. Make the lesson fun and engaging by creating the plan with kids.

What You'll Need	All Ages	Babies	Toddlers	Preschoolers	School-Age Children
Paper and pencil	🖐				
Stopwatch	🖐				

Fire officials agree that parents should begin teaching fire safety when their children are very young. As a group, parents can work with their children to take the following steps to create a fire safety plan. Please know some of the items must be completed at their own homes:

1. **Discuss smoke alarms.**
   Gather near a smoke alarm in your home and explain to children that the device makes a loud noise when it detects smoke. The noise alerts people to follow the fire safety plan and leave the home quickly. If appropriate, press the test button on the alarm to emit the noise. (The U.S. Fire Administration recommends familiarizing all your children with the sound of a smoke alarm, but use your discretion for the little ones since it can be quite loud. We'd suggest putting the baby in another room and having toddlers block their ears.) Children can then help make sure your home has enough smoke alarms in working order. For example,

preschoolers can check that a smoke alarm is on each level of the home and in each bedroom. If not, make a plan to install smoke alarms as soon as possible.

2. **Draw a map to safety.**
   If your home is on fire, how will you escape? By following a map! Help school-age children draw a map of the layout of their home, including all the rooms, doors, and windows. When the map is complete, they should review it with their family. Then go to each child's bedroom and discuss two different ways to exit the room and the home. Children can each use a finger to trace the two quickest routes from the bedroom to the nearest exterior door. Mark these routes on the map.

3. **Choose a meeting spot.**
   Together with their family, kids should choose a designated "meeting spot" a safe distance outside the home. Explain to children this is where you will meet if there's a fire and you all need to exit the house. A toddler can help make this decision. Give him two appropriate choices and let him decide.

4. **Practice crawling!**
   Show children how they should crawl on their hands and knees or on their bellies when escaping the house during a fire. Explain how staying low lets them breathe the air and not the smoke floating above.

   Also show them what to do if their clothing catches on fire: They must *stop* whatever they're doing, *drop* to the ground, and *roll* to extinguish the flames. All children will have fun practicing this drill, even a baby! Place her on her back and roll her carefully and slowly from side to side (but not all the way over).

5. Have a fire drill.
   After doing the tasks above, all the children can participate in a fire drill! Have children go to one or more rooms (depending on children's age) and tell them to be ready to follow the fire safety plan when they hear the "smoke alarm." Make a loud beeping sound to simulate the smoke alarm, then start a stopwatch to time the drill. Encourage children to crawl quickly but calmly out of the house and quickly walk to the meeting spot outside. At one point, tell them to stop, drop, and roll. When everyone is at the meeting spot, stop the stopwatch and record the time it took to complete the drill. If the kids like, go ahead and do the drill again, and challenge them to beat the previous drill's time.

Host Tip
Encourage each family to make copies of their maps and post them on the inside of every bedroom door. Families should practice the drill often in the future in their own homes.

A Royal Birthday Throne

This easy-to-do project is a great way to make playmates feel like kings and queens on their birthdays!

What You'll Need	All Ages	Babies	Toddlers	Preschoolers	School-Age Children
Decoration supplies, such as streamers, paper, tape, crayons, stickers, tempera paint, child-safe scissors, and so on	✋				

On each child's birthday, let the other children make a throne so the birthday child can receive the royal treatment. Choose a chair appropriate for the birthday child, then give other children various supplies to decorate the chair. If they need direction, prompt them to consider the birthday child's favorite colors, cartoon characters, or nursery rhymes as decoration ideas. Below are some age-appropriate suggestions for how each child can help decorate the throne. (We strongly advise not using balloons for this activity. They pose a serious choking risk to children.)

Babies

Babies can add the perfect decoration for a playmate's birthday throne: If a friend is turning three, paint and press three of the baby's fingers onto a piece of paper. If a friend is turning eight, use eight fingers. You can cut out the imprint and glue this decoration to the throne.

Toddlers

Tear off twelve-inch pieces of streamer for toddlers to decorate. Lay them on the table and tape down the ends. Toddlers can cover the pieces with stickers, then help you attach them to the birthday child's chair. Let them decide where they should go.

Preschoolers

What is the birthday child's favorite activity or animal? How about a favorite food or friend? Have preschoolers draw pictures of the favorite things to tape to the birthday child's chair.

School-Age Children

School-age children can print the birthday child's name in fancy lettering or write a special birthday message on a sheet of paper, then tape it to the back of the chair.

Host Tip

If possible, try to make the throne a surprise for the birthday child. Have friends decorate the chair beforehand! You may also want to create a special crown for the birthday child (see "King and Queen Crowns" on page 312).

Time Capsule

Create a time capsule to capture this time in the children's lives!

What You'll Need	All Ages	Babies	Toddlers	Preschoolers	School-Age Children
Plastic, metal, or heavy-duty rubber container (roughly the size of an adult shoebox)	🖐				
Roll of ribbon	🖐				
Bathroom scale	🖐				
Index cards	🖐				
Marker	🖐				
Photos, drawings, or other mementos	🖐				

Explain to the children that a time capsule is something in which to store fun and unique mementos that describe what a person or community is like right now. On a certain date in the future, you will open the time capsule and see how much things have changed! To get started, choose a small container as your capsule, then work with the children to create special mementos. Below you'll find some recommendations.

After your time capsule is full of mementos, seal it and decide together when it will be reopened. Kids grow and change quickly, but at least several months should pass so the children can easily see how much they've changed since making the time capsule. The longer you wait, the more dramatic the changes will be. Once you choose a reopening date, tell them you will store it in an out-of-the-way place until then. We recommend in your attic, basement, or garage. (Just make sure to write down its location!)

Height and Weight
Use a roll of ribbon to measure each child's height from head to toe. Cut the ribbon and write the child's name on it. Use a bathroom scale to record children's weights on separate index cards.

Special Skills or Characteristics
Record children's latest skills or characteristics on separate index cards. For example, record how high toddlers can count and how many teeth a baby has. Also record what makes each child unique, such as "He laughs when Daddy scratches his belly!"

Favorites
Record children's favorite toys, songs, stories, food, or other items on separate index cards. Preschoolers may enjoy drawing pictures of the favorites on the cards.

Handprint
Trace each child's hand on construction paper. If you like, cut out the tracings and let children decorate the cutouts with crayons. Be sure to label each with the date and appropriate name.

Other Mementos
Include other special items like drawings or photos. School-age children may choose to include an assignment or test from school.

Host Tip
Put a copy of the daily paper in the time capsule. It will be interesting later to see what the big news were on the day you made the capsule.

Show-and-Tell Me

Let children show their pride and knowledge with a rousing round of show-and-tell.

What You'll Need	All Ages	Babies	Toddlers	Preschoolers	School-Age Children
Special objects	✋				
Timer	✋				

Invite children to each bring a special object for show-and-tell with their playmates. It may be a toy, book, souvenir, art project, or collectible. You should grab an object, too. Gather in a circle. To demonstrate how to "show-and-tell," hold up your object for everyone to see, then tell them about where you got it and why it's so special to you. Have children take turns showing and telling about their special objects.

Babies

When it's baby's turn to show, let her show off a new skill. For example, has she learned sign language? Can she smile on cue? Blow a raspberry? Sit up on her own or pick up a piece of cereal? For the "telling" part, a parent or older child can share memories of when baby first began doing the particular skill, and how it compares with other siblings in their family.

Toddlers
Ask toddlers to demonstrate ways they play with, use, or enjoy their objects. Encourage them to tell everyone about their special objects by asking a few yes-or-no questions. For example, "Do you love that toy?" "Do you sleep with that toy?"

Preschoolers
Preschoolers will have no problem showing off their special objects and telling their playmates all about them. When it's a playmate's turn, however, teach preschoolers how to be good listeners and encourage them to ask thoughtful questions. Model this behavior by asking the speaker, "You mentioned that someone who is very special bought this bear for you. Who is that special person?" Then prompt preschoolers by saying, "Did your friend mention something you want to hear more about?"

School-Age Children
For a twist on show-and-tell, challenge school-age children to show off skills they can do, then tell their playmates how to do it. For example, if they play soccer, they can show moves with a soccer ball, then teach playmates how to do the tricks.

Friendship Fun Jar

Your playgroup will never run out of ideas for fun with this activity!

What You'll Need	All Ages	Babies	Toddlers	Preschoolers	School-Age Children
Large sheet of paper	✋				
Crayons	✋				
Magazines, child-safe scissors, and glue sticks			✋		
Medium-size jar	✋				

Write each child's name at the top of a large sheet of paper. Together, think of some fun ways to spend time together (see age-appropriate suggestions below). Write each idea under the appropriate child's name. If you like, older children can transfer each idea to index cards and draw pictures of the ideas (or glue magazine images that depict them) as visual cues for the younger children. Then place all the ideas in a jar so you can pick one at future playdates.

Babies

Older playmates will have to help come up with fun ways to spend time with a baby. They may suggest storytime or a field trip to the zoo as something the youngest playmates enjoy. Have them share their ideas with the baby, who will love the attention from playmates.

Toddlers

Toddlers will likely benefit from some visual cues during the brainstorming of ideas. Flip through a magazine to look for kids having fun. What are they drawn to? What makes them smile? During the brainstorming, encourage toddlers to clap when they hear an idea they love.

Preschoolers

Preschoolers can help come up with ideas for fun. Give them each a chance to share details of their favorite things to do, such as dancing or playing a favorite board game.

School-Age Children

School-age children can use this opportunity to think of new ways to spend time with their friends. Is there a hobby they would love to introduce to others? Is there a place in town they love to go? Consider this an 'active' show-and-tell opportunity.

Host Tip

Make sure your friend fun jar includes a good dose of physical activities. Suggest a scavenger hunt outside or a game of Wiffle ball.

Get-Well Basket

Have children cheer up a sick friend with a thoughtful get-well basket.

What You'll Need	All Ages	Babies	Toddlers	Preschoolers	School-Age Children
Basket	🖐				
Basket goodies (see next page for examples)	🖐				
Cotton blanket	🖐				
Fabric markers	🖐				
Ribbon	🖐				

Show playmates an empty basket and tell them they're going to fill it with goodies that will cheer up a friend when he isn't feeling well. Have children use their imaginations to decide what goodies to include in the basket. Ask them what things would make them feel better if they were sick. Challenge them to come up with ideas any friend of any age will appreciate, or encourage them to have a balance of items for younger and older friends. If they need direction, suggest the ideas on the next page.

After deciding what goodies to include, have kids collect the items, then help you arrange them in the basket. Next, have children decorate a small cotton blanket with fabric markers. You can trace a baby's hand on the blanket, a toddler can doodle on it, preschoolers can draw a smiley face, and school-age children can write well-wishes or a comforting message. When the ink is dry, wrap the blanket around the basket, tie it closed with a ribbon, and store the basket. Plan to present the basket whenever one of the playmates is sick.

Host Tip
Remind children that the items in the basket will be stored away until someone is sick. Therefore, they shouldn't include items they use or want on a regular basis, such as a beloved toy or frequently watched DVD.

Basket Goodies
Tissues
Plush animal
Quiet toy
CD of relaxing music
Special DVD
Coloring book and crayons

Bell: The sick friend can ring the bell from his bed or the couch when he needs something. (See "Ring Those Bells" on page 117 for a homemade variety.)

IOUs: Sick kids always feel like they're missing out on things. With these IOUs, children can give a sick friend something to look forward to when he feels better. They can write "IOU a game of tag" or "IOU a chance to borrow one of my toys."

Chapter 8

World Friends

I took out a map the other day to show my kids where I was heading on a business trip. "We're here," I said, pointing to Massachusetts. "And I'm going here." I moved my finger over a few inches to point to Arkansas. They looked puzzled, as I knew they would. Finally, my son asked, "But why do you even have to take a plane there?"

—Heather

Most children don't realize there's a big, wide world beyond their own horizon. They also don't realize their actions can make this world a better place. In this chapter, children will learn about different lands, cultures, and languages. Most importantly, they'll also learn about contributing to the world in special ways by showing compassion and respect for all living things. It's never too early to expand children's view.

Hello and Goodbye!

Introduce new cultures to children through different languages!

What You'll Need	All Ages	Babies	Toddlers	Preschoolers	School-Age Children
Plush animal			🖐		
World atlas or globe				🖐	🖐

Young children learn foreign languages quicker than teens and adults. Teach children how to say "Hello" and "Goodbye" in different languages. See next page for a list of these words and their pronunciations. Feel free to add other languages to your list. If some children are learning a foreign language at school, encourage them to teach their playmates other simple words in that language.

Babies

Waving "bye-bye" is one of the first gestures babies learn. Show a baby how to wave goodbye in another language. For example, make eye contact, then wave your hand while saying, "*Adiós!*" or, "*Sayonara!*"

Toddlers

Play a fun game with toddlers to help them learn foreign words. Hold a plush animal in front of them. As you hide it from view, say, "Goodbye" in one of the languages. Then say, "Hello," in that language while quickly bringing the animal back into view. Do these actions again and again, encouraging toddlers to say the appropriate words. They may not pronounce them correctly, but they'll enjoy saying them as part of the game.

Preschoolers and School-Age Children

Teach older children the foreign words on the list, then use this activity to strengthen geography and role-playing skills. Provide a world atlas or globe and point to a country whose people speak that language. For example, point to France and say to one child, "Pretend you're buying bread from your friend the baker. What will you say to each other?" Encourage the children to say the appropriate foreign words during the scene. For example, one child can say to a friend, "*Bonjour*! I would like to buy some bread."

Hello and *Goodbye* in Other Languages		
Language	Hello (Pronunciation)	Goodbye (Pronunciation)
Chinese	*Ni hao* (NEE-how)	*Zaijian* (dzeye-zhee-EN)
French	*Bonjour* (bone-ZHOOR)	*Au revior* (oh reh-VWAHR)
German	*Guten Tag* (GOO-tun tahk)	*Auf Wiedersehen* (owf VEE-der-zayn)
Italian	*Buon giorno* (bwone JOHR-noh)	*Arrivederci* (ah-ree-vah-DARE-chee)
Japanese	*Domo* (DOH-moh)	*Sayonara* (sigh-yoh-NAH-rah)
Spanish	*Buenos dias* (bway-nohs DEE-ahs)	*Adiós* (ah-DYOHS)
Swedish	*God dag* (goo dog)	*Adjö* (ahd-YOH)

Feed All the Little Birds

Children can take care of their feathered friends with these simple birdfeeders.

What You'll Need	All Ages	Babies	Toddlers	Preschoolers	School-Age Children
Round cereal with holes, like Cheerios or Froot Loops	🖐				
Bowls			🖐	🖐	🖐
Pipe cleaners	🖐				
Yarn and scissors			🖐	🖐	🖐

Pour the cereal into separate bowls. Show the group how to string the cereal onto a pipe cleaner to make a hanging bird-feeder. When done, twist each end of the pipe cleaner into a loop. Then use yarn to tie the birdfeeders to the branches of nearby trees.

Babies

If the baby is eating cereal, place a few pieces on a highchair tray and let her practice grasping them. She'll see her friends working with the cereal, so she'll want to pick it up, too. If the baby isn't eating solids yet, rub a pipe cleaner on the soles of her feet for a fuzzy sensation!

Toddlers

This activity is a perfect chance for toddlers to work on their small-motor skills, like picking up a small cereal piece and stringing it onto the pipe cleaner. Have them hang their birdfeeder near a window in their home, if possible. They'll enjoy watching the birds eat their work.

Preschoolers

Give preschoolers colorful cereal to string onto their pipe cleaner. Show them how they can make patterns with the pieces. For example, they can string on a blue piece, then a red one, then a blue one, and so on. Encourage them to come up with patterns of their own.

School-Age Children

School-age children may enjoy making several birdfeeders in different patterns. Encourage them to join their birdfeeders together to create a figure or design to display from a tree branch.

👣 Did You Know?

Birds use a lot of energy while flying, and many species eat up to 100 percent of their body weight each day to power their flight.

A Birdbath Haven

Birds need reliable access to clean, fresh water, especially in hot weather, so create a homemade birdbath.

What You'll Need	All Ages	Babies	Toddlers	Preschoolers	School-Age Children
Old sheet	✋				
Scissors	✋				
Sponges	✋				
Acrylic paint	✋				
3 medium-size clay pots and a large clay saucer (available at gardening stores)	✋				
Paper bowls	✋				
Small tin baking dish		✋			
Bucket			✋		
Small plastic toy insects	✋				
Ceramic glue	✋				
Bird guide					✋

On a sunny day, lay an old sheet out in the yard for your workspace. Cut sponges into small squares and pour paint into a few paper bowls. Children can use the sponges to paint three clay pots and the outside of a large clay saucer. (Only the outsides of the pots will be visible in the end.) When the paint is dry, you and any older children can assemble the pieces into a birdbath, while younger children help put on the final touches (see each age group below). Place the finished birdbath within view of a window, then watch for birds to take a dip!

Babies

While playmates create the birdbath, a baby can enjoy playing in his own "birdbath." If the baby can sit up on his own, pour some water into a small tin baking dish and let him explore it with his hands. Only use as much water as you are willing to let him get wet! If the baby isn't sitting up yet, hold the dish for him or dab some water on his bare toes with a sponge.

Toddlers

Toddlers will enjoy painting with sponges. While the paint dries, assign them to find small rocks to add to the saucer. Have them wash the rocks in a bucket of water before placing them in the birdbath.

Preschoolers

When the birdbath is assembled, preschoolers can help decorate it with plastic insects. They can show you where to glue the insects onto the pots. They can also fill the birdbath with water and make sure it always has a fresh supply.

School-Age Children

School-age children can help you assemble the birdbath: Turn one pot upside down. On top of that pot, glue another pot right side up. Then glue the third pot upside down on top of the second pot. Finally, glue the saucer right side up on top of the last pot. When birds begin to visit the birdbath, school-age children can use a bird guide to identify each species.

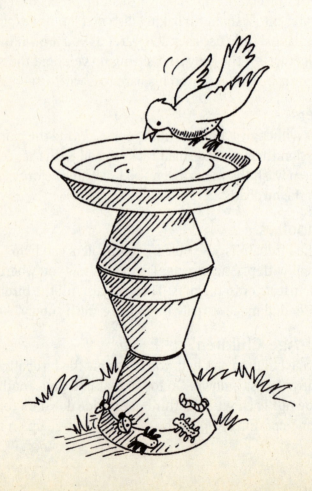

Moving around the World

Tour the world's landscapes with this fun action song!

What You'll Need	All Ages	Babies	Toddlers	Preschoolers	School-Age Children
Voices and bodies!	✋				

In a room with plenty of open space, sing and act out the following song with children to the tune of "The Mulberry Bush." Each verse describes a different landscape from around the world.

Here we fly 'round the flat grasslands,
the flat grasslands, the flat grasslands.
Here we fly 'round the flat grasslands
where it is so windy.

(Spin, walk fast, and wave your arms as if being pushed by the wind.)

Here we skate on the polar ice,
the polar ice, the polar ice.
Here we skate on the polar ice
where it is so chilly.

(Move your feet in a skating motion and rub your arms as if cold.)

Here we slide down the sandy dunes,
the sandy dunes, the sandy dunes.
Here we slide down the sandy dunes
in the dry, hot desert.

(Roll on the floor.)

Here we climb the great big trees,

the great big trees, the great big trees.
Here we climb the great big trees
in the evergreen forest.

(Move arms to act out climbing while marching.)

Here we run up the tall mountains,
the tall mountains, the tall mountains.
Here we run up the tall mountains
so we can reach the sky.

(Run in exaggerated motion while reaching arms toward the sky.)

Babies and Toddlers

You can hold the baby in your arms during this activity and move her body as directed in the song. She'll love listening to her playmates sing and watching them act out the movements! Toddlers will likely be a beat behind the others as they mimic the older kids' actions, but that's okay. They'll enjoy doing the movements on their own.

Preschoolers and School-Age Children

Preschoolers and school-age children can take turns leading the movements to act out. Challenge them to think of other landscapes to add to the song. For example, they can come up with actions to do on an oceanfront or in a valley.

Adopt a Tree

Have children adopt a special tree in your yard or neighborhood. They'll learn a valuable lesson about the beauty of nature.

What You'll Need	All Ages	Babies	Toddlers	Preschoolers	School-Age Children
A picnic (see "Packin' a Picnic" on page 19 for ideas)	✋				

Prepare a picnic with the group, then take a walk in your yard or in your neighborhood, and together select a tree to "adopt." Sit by the tree and observe its beauty. Ask the children to describe its leaves, trunk, height, and so on. Enjoy the picnic under the foliage. Together, make plans to visit this special tree regularly.

Babies and Toddlers

Babies and toddlers will enjoy being outside with friends, and their adopted tree will delight their senses. Gently stroke a leaf on the baby's cheek. Encourage toddlers to touch the tree bark with their hands.

Preschoolers and School-Age Children

Help preschoolers and school-age children identify the type of tree you've adopted. Discuss the different ways trees benefit the environment. For example, trees provide shade and shelter to various animals. They also help protect against soil erosion and offset carbon dioxide emissions—important concepts you can begin to explain to children.

Host Tip

For added enjoyment, read *The Giving Tree* by Shel Silverstein to the children while sitting under your adopted tree. Afterward, ask them why the tree in the story was so giving. Tell them that by adopting a tree, they're also being giving.

In addition to visiting your adopted tree, you may also want to care for it. (Be sure to ask permission before tending to a neighborhood tree outside your property.) Here are some ways you can care for your adopted tree. Perhaps the group will brainstorm other ideas. Caring for the tree will help develop their nurturing skills as well as help protect the environment!

- Pull weeds from around the trunk and pack fresh soil around the base.
- Water your tree.
- Plant flowers at the base.
- Chart your tree's growth by periodically taking a photo in front of it.
- Attract feathered friends to your tree by hanging birdfeeders from its branches. (See page 266.)

One group of friends named their "friendship" trees. One was called Maple and the other Syrup!

—Lisa

Recycling Center

The average American generates more than four pounds of trash every day. That's a lot of garbage! Recycling helps reduce waste and conserve materials, so make a recycling center in your home.

What You'll Need	All Ages	Babies	Toddlers	Preschoolers	School-Age Children
Marker	✋				
3 boxes	✋				
Duct tape	✋				
Old magazines			✋	✋	✋
Child-safe scissors			✋	✋	✋
Glue stick			✋	✋	✋
3 paper bags	✋				
Uncooked beans		✋			
Empty water bottle		✋			

Have older children help you label three boxes *Paper*, *Plastic*, and *Glass*. They can then add visual cues by cutting out magazine images of recyclable items and gluing them onto the appropriate boxes. Attach the boxes in a row with tape, then place a paper grocery bag in each box. Explain to the children that it's everyone's responsibility to place recyclable items in the appropriate bags rather than throwing them in the regular garbage. Also explain that when the bags are full you will remove them from the boxes and set them out for collection or bring them to a drop-off site.

Babies

While his older playmates work on the recycling center, make a recycled rattle to keep the baby occupied. Place uncooked beans in an empty water bottle. Be sure to secure the cap tightly. The baby will enjoy shaking, banging, and rolling his new toy. If he's younger, shake and roll the rattle for him. He'll enjoy listening to the sound.

Toddlers, Preschoolers, and School-Age Children

Older children can team up to decorate the boxes. School-age children can lead the project by finding images of paper, plastic, and glass items commonly found in a house. Preschoolers can then cut the images and add glue to their backs. Finally, toddlers can stick the images onto the appropriate boxes, with help. When they're done, send them on a search around the home for any recyclables they can add to the bags right away, such as yesterday's newspaper, an empty soda bottle on the counter, or a near-empty jam jar in the fridge. Help them wash out the items then determine in which bag they each belong.

Host Tip
Remind children that the home recycling center is a prime location for arts-and-crafts supplies. With activities such as "Recyclables" on page 333, children can learn how to "recycle" the items to create artwork or practical items.

Charity Roundup

Introduce children to the satisfaction of helping others in need.

What You'll Need	All Ages	Babies	Toddlers	Preschoolers	School-Age Children
Donation items (see below)	🖐				
Boxes	🖐				
Blanket		🖐			
Paper towels, tape, glue, and child-safe scissors					🖐
Paper and pencil					🖐

Before the playdate, ask the group to gather toys, plush animals, books, games, and clothing that they've outgrown or no longer want. Once together, explain in simple terms what you will do with the items. For example: "Won't it be nice to give these things you've outgrown to children who need them?" Older kids can help you sort and box the items, then choose a charitable organization where you can donate them. Congratulate them for giving to others! (To avoid future tears of regret, don't let children donate any beloved belongings. Thank them for their generosity, but suggest other toys to donate.)

Babies

A baby older than six months can help pack up the items—and practice her ability to grasp and release. Give her an object she can grab and hold, like a plush animal, and encourage her to release it into a box. A baby younger than six months can enjoy some tummy time while her friends work: Lay her on a blanket with a few plush animals nearby. The furry friends may inspire to her exercise her neck muscles to get a look at them.

Toddlers

Play a roundup game with toddlers using the donation items. Describe an object and ask them to get it and drop it in the box. For example, say, "I'm thinking of a toy that's soft and blue. It has a ribbon around its neck. Can you bring that toy to the box?" This exercise will develop their listening skills as well as their vocabulary.

Preschoolers

Challenge preschoolers' categorizing skills with a fun activity. Have them sort the items into categories, such as things you wear, things you play with, and all other things. Or have them sort the items by the charities that will receive them. For example, tell them baby items go to one charity, older children's clothing goes to another, and toys go to a third. When they're finished sorting, have them put the items from each category into a separate box.

School-Age Children

Because donation items must be in good condition, let school-age children inspect each item and clean it and make minor repairs as needed. Give them tools like damp and dry paper towels, tape, glue, and scissors. If an item needs fixing beyond their abilities, have them write a "work order" for you. For example, "Please sew on the bear's eye," or, "This shirt has a stain."

Host Tip

Research local establishments or national charities that accept donations in your area. Here are some ideas:

- Libraries
- Food shelves
- Places of worship
- Shelters
- Hospitals
- Charitable organizations, such as:
  - The Salvation Army (http://www.salvationarmyusa.org)
  - The Home for Little Wanderers (http://www.thehome.org)
  - Goodwill Industries International, Inc. (http://www.goodwill.org)
  - Newborns in Need (http://www.newbornsinneed.org)

Fashion from around the World

Learn about places with different climates, cultures, and traditions by creating these easy-to-make fashions!

What You'll Need	All Ages	Babies	Toddlers	Preschoolers	School-Age Children
World atlas or globe	🖐				
Bath towels		🖐			
Old bath towels			🖐		
Scissors			🖐		
Beach towels				🖐	🖐

Explain to the group that different people wear different clothing all around the world. On an atlas or globe, point out the following places: Java, Brazil, Alaska, and India. Talk about the different climates and cultures in these places and how that might affect people's clothing. Then tell the children they're going to create fashions from each of those places. Help children create their garments, then have them take turns modeling and describing the clothing to one another. Encourage children to ask questions about their playmates' garments. For example, "Is that comfortable to wear?" Ask them to compare the clothing to the clothing they wear in this country.

Babies

People in Java wear a sarong, a large sheet of fabric wrapped around the waist and worn as a skirt. Use a bath towel to create a sarong on a baby. He may not tolerate wearing the garment for long, so be sure he's first to display the fashion to his playmates!

Toddlers

People in Brazil, especially ranchers, wear ponchos. Make ponchos for toddlers by cutting out a large circle in the center of each old bath towel. Slide it over their heads and have them pretend to be ranchers galloping around on horses.

Preschoolers

Alaskan Native people often wear parkas, which are jackets made from animal fur. To create parkas for preschoolers, wrap a towel over their shoulders and loosely tie a knot to hold it together. Then wrap and tie another towel over their heads to make a hood. Centuries ago, people believed that when they wore a parka, they took on the characteristics of the animals from which it was constructed. Encourage preschoolers to act like an Alaskan fur animal, such as a wolf or a mink.

School-Age Children

Women in India often wear a sari. Have school-age children create this garment by wrapping one end of a beach towel around their waist and draping the other end over their head or one shoulder. Have them walk in the garment—it'll be good practice for posture and balance! Men in India sometimes wear a traditional garment called a *lungi* (pronounced "loon-gee"), a cloth that's draped around the waist. If you like, have school-age children create and wear that garment.

Host Tip
This activity is a prime photo opportunity. Have a camera nearby to capture the fashions!

Chapter 9

Arts & Crafts

Nearly every inch of my refrigerator door is covered with crayon drawings, glitter-strewn construction paper, and painted handprints. When I have a moment to pause before opening the door, I admire my children's creativity and marvel at how they interpret their world.

—Heather

Children express their creativity as they work side by side on arts-and-crafts projects. In this chapter, children will discover their own artistic talents as well as one another's. Because art projects can get complicated and messy, we've kept things simple. These activities—which include paper-plate self-portraits, water-bottle aquariums, and finger-paint color wheels—often use the same materials for children of all ages, and we've included specific instructions to bring out the artist in every age group.

Let Me See Your Funny Face

Let the children see all the silly and interesting things they can do with their faces!

What You'll Need	All Ages	Babies	Toddlers	Preschoolers	School-Age Children
Large mirror	🖐				
Old magazines		🖐			🖐
Child-safe scissors			🖐	🖐	🖐
Colored construction paper			🖐	🖐	🖐
Glue stick			🖐	🖐	🖐
Paper plates			🖐	🖐	🖐
Stapler					🖐

Gather the playmates around a large mirror to make funny faces and admire their similar and unique features. Then older children can create self-portraits by gluing construction paper features onto paper plates.

Babies

Babies will enjoy studying their faces in the mirror. Touch their noses and eyes as they gaze at themselves. This action will help them learn that the reflection in the mirror is theirs. To strengthen neck muscles, place babies on their tummies in front of the mirror—they'll work hard to get a good look at themselves. While their playmates make funny faces in the mirror, babies may even try to mimic them. For more fun, flip through magazines that have lots of close-up photos of faces for them to admire and study.

Toddlers
Have toddlers identify the different features of their faces, including the colors of their eyes and hair. Cut out sets of eyes, noses, mouths, and hair for them from construction paper. Help toddlers glue the cutouts onto a paper plate to create self-portraits.

Preschoolers
Preschoolers can cut out sets of eyes, noses, mouths, and hair from construction paper for their self-portraits. They may also want to include other facial details like eyebrows, eyelashes, and ears. Preschoolers understand different feelings, too. They may want to create a happy, silly, or tired face. While they work on the project, ask them to identify how they look similar to or different from their playmates.

School-Age Children
School-age children can also use photos from magazines to create a more intricate or silly self-portrait. They can cut out eyes, noses, and mouths from images in the magazine. Encourage them to create portraits of their playmates, too, and then staple the paper plates together side by side for a homemade group portrait.

Trace a Place Mat

These fun and functional place mats will teach children about the objects they need before sitting down for a meal.

What You'll Need	All Ages	Babies	Toddlers	Preschoolers	School-Age Children
Construction paper	✋				
Child-safe scissors	✋				
Glue sticks	✋				
Plastic plates and cups	✋				
Age-appropriate eating utensils	✋				
Crayons	✋				
Magazines or supermarket circulars				✋	

Trace a plate, a cup, and eating utensils onto a sheet of construction paper for each toddler. Preschoolers and school-age children may do this task independently. Older children can cut out their own shapes and glue them onto other sheets of construction paper in the correct places.

Babies

You or older children can make special place mats for babies to explore. After tracing the objects, draw some happy faces on the tracings. For a fun hide-and-seek game, place a plastic plate, cup, and spoon on the correct spaces and see if the babies can find the smiling faces by moving the objects around. For babies younger than six months, playmates can remove the objects while saying, "Peekaboo!"

Toddlers

Trace the cutouts onto a blank sheet of construction paper in the proper places for a matching game. Challenge toddlers to compare the cutouts with the tracings on the paper, and then ask the toddlers to match them up. Use verbal prompts such as, "Wow, this is a big circle. Can you find another big circle in front of you?" Glue the cutouts onto the place mats as they make matches.

Preschoolers

Demonstrate how preschoolers can use one hand to hold an object steady and the other hand to trace the object with a crayon. Along with cutting, tracing is a great way to further develop motor skills.

School-Age Children

After gluing their shapes onto their place mats, school-age children may enjoy adding colorful food cutouts from magazines or supermarket circulars. They can depict their favorite meals (like pizza and milk).

Host Tip
Put these place mats on the table before mealtime. Older children can use them as a guide to set the table.

Squeeze-Me Sponge Art

In this activity, kids will work with the texture of sponges to create wonderful art!

What You'll Need	All Ages	Babies	Toddlers	Preschoolers	School-Age Children
Child-safe scissors			✋	✋	✋
New sponges			✋	✋	✋
Facecloth		✋			
Small baking pans	✋				
Washable tempera paint			✋	✋	✋
Sheets of paper			✋	✋	✋
Stapler				✋	

To get started, you or school-age children can cut shapes like stars, circles, and squares from new sponges.

Babies

With babies in highchairs, pour a bit of water into a small baking pan and set it on their trays. Sponges may be a choking hazard, so give them facecloths to explore instead. For babies six months or older, show them how to dip the facecloth into the water and squeeze it out. This sensation will delight them as they build small-motor skills and the muscles in their hands. For babies younger than six months, rub the damp cloth on their cheeks. They'll enjoy feeling the new texture.

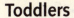

Toddlers

Sponges may be a new art medium for toddlers. Show them how to dip their sponge shape into a baking pan of paint and then press it onto a sheet of paper for a colorful shape collage. This activity is a great chance to review the names of different shapes and colors.

Preschoolers

Preschoolers can create a shape-counting book. Label separate sheets of paper *Circle*, *Square*, and *Triangle* and encourage the children to put only the correct sponge shape on the corresponding sheet of paper. This activity aids in word recognition. Once the paint dries, have them count the circles on the circle page and write the number on that page. Do the same for every shape page and then staple the pages together. This will be a great book for them to share with their playmates.

School-Age Children

School-age children can create objects or scenes with the sponge shapes. Perhaps they will paint a starry night, using the square and rectangle for a house and the stars for the sky. You can tap into their creative sides by suggesting they make abstract art shapes or patterns.

Host Tip
Have children help with cleanup. They can wash the table or the baking pans with a clean sponge. Babies may mimic them by wiping their highchair trays.

Look at Us Now Murals

Using teamwork, children can create their own life-size body murals.

What You'll Need	All Ages	Babies	Toddlers	Preschoolers	School-Age Children
Butcher paper (or paper grocery bags taped together)	🖐				
Crayons	🖐				
Tape			🖐		
Mirror				🖐	
Child-safe scissors					🖐

Each child can take a turn lying on a piece of butcher paper while you or playmates trace their bodies with a crayon. There are sure to be some tickle spots along the way!

Babies

It may be difficult for babies to remain still as playmates trace around them. Try laying babies on their bellies, sides, or backs on the butcher paper. Let the babies move as they want and trace any pose they make.

Toddlers

Toddlers may prefer standing while being traced. Tape the paper to the wall and have them stand with their backs against it. When the tracing is complete, they will be impressed by their life-size body outline. Have them identify their body parts by asking, "Where are your legs? Where is your belly?" and so on. As you (or an older playmate) help them add features with crayons, prompt them by asking, "Where should your eyes go?"

Preschoolers

If preschoolers help trace their playmates, encourage them to keep their crayons close to the bodies being traced so their tracings are accurate. When they decorate their own body murals, have them look in the mirror so they can identify which crayons to use to color their hair, eyes, and clothes. They may decide to dress their body mural as a superhero or ballerina.

School-Age Children

Challenge school-age children to imitate Pablo Picasso, one of the most important artists of the twentieth century. Much of his work involved colorful collages of mismatched objects. For instance, school-age children can trace a playmate's hand, cut out the tracing, and use it as one of their hands in their body mural. They can also color their features in mismatching colors.

> **Did You Know?**
> By the time Pablo Picasso died at age ninety-two, he had created twenty-two thousand works of art in a variety of mediums, including sculpture, ceramics, mosaics, stage design, and graphic arts.

Host Tip
Have the artists take their body murals home to display in their rooms.

Portable Seas

Create a mesmerizing, portable sea using water bottles, trinkets, and a little imagination.

What You'll Need	All Ages	Babies	Toddlers	Preschoolers	School-Age Children
Clear plastic water bottles, ¾ full, with caps	👋				
Blue food coloring	👋				
Red and yellow food coloring					👋
1 teaspoon vegetable oil per bottle					👋
"Sea" objects, like hermit crabs (small acorns or rocks), minnows (small, twisted strips of aluminum foil), sea-floor rocks (pebbles), fish (sequins), and dolphins (small pieces of drinking straws)	👋				
Glue	👋				

Begin by removing the bottle labels and adding a few drops of blue food coloring to the water with older children's help. While preschoolers and school-age children add "sea objects" to their bottles, younger children can watch as you add objects to theirs. When portable seas are completed, use glue to secure the caps to the bottles.

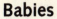

Babies

Babies will enjoy watching as objects are dropped into portable seas. When done, place the bottle in front of the baby on the floor and gently push the bottle so it rolls away. If babies are six months or older, this action may entice them to retrieve the bottle. If babies are younger than six months, hold the bottle close to their ears and tilt it gently back and forth to create waves. The sound may remind them of the womb. To visually stimulate them, hold the bottle in front of them and encourage them to watch the sea objects float back and forth.

Toddlers

Let toddlers point to the objects they want you to add to their bottles. As you drop each one into the water, playfully say, "We're going to pretend this is a hermit crab." Talk about the sea with the toddlers. Ask, "Who lives in the sea? How do they get around?" When you're done, they will love using their hands to shake the bottle as hard as they can.

Preschoolers

Preschoolers will enjoy watching the food coloring mix with the water, and they'll have fun shaking up their seas after they have added their objects. This activity can also be calming once the shaking stops. They may become entranced as they watch the objects slowly settle in the bottle.

School-Age Children

School-age children may want a blue sea, but as a variation, give them food coloring in all three primary colors at the beginning of the activity. Ask them to drip two colors into their water bottle and have them predict what color they will create. For instance, blue and red creates purple. Yellow and red makes orange. Before they choose their sea objects, ask them to predict which will float and which will sink. Were their predictions correct? They can also add a teaspoon of vegetable oil to their bottles. The oil will float to the top, giving their portable sea the look of a lava lamp.

Host Tip
The portable sea is a great toy during bath time, car rides, or walks in the stroller.

Wild Wheel of Color

Finger paints offer a chance for the kids to use their favorite art accessories—their hands! In this activity, children will learn how colors mix together to create new ones.

What You'll Need	All Ages	Babies	Toddlers	Preschoolers	School-Age Children
Paper plates			🖐	🖐	🖐
Pencil			🖐	🖐	🖐
Finger paints in primary colors			🖐	🖐	🖐
Paper			🖐	🖐	🖐
Smocks (or old T-shirts)			🖐	🖐	🖐
Wet wipes	🖐				
Newspaper			🖐	🖐	🖐
Plain yogurt		🖐			
Food coloring		🖐			
Wax paper		🖐			

On each paper plate, draw six wedges of equal size, as though slicing a pizza. On every other wedge, dab a bit of paint in this color order: red, blue, yellow. Instruct toddlers, preschoolers, and school-age children to dip their fingers in red and blue finger paint and mix the two together in the blank space between those two colors on their paper plates. Have them do the same for the spaces between the blue and yellow wedges and the yellow and red wedges. When done, they will have a color wheel: red, purple, blue, green, yellow, and orange. Use the wheels to make finger-paint creations on a separate sheet of paper.

Note: This activity may be messy, so put smocks or old T-shirts on the children beforehand and have plenty of wet wipes handy to clean up messy fingers when you're done. It's also a good idea to lay newspaper under each child's sheet of paper, and on the floor under the table.

Babies
Babies love to explore with their hands and mouths, so if any babies are eating dairy, make a batch of yogurt "paint" they can enjoy while their playmates enjoy their finger paint. Mix plain yogurt with food coloring and place it on a piece of wax paper on their highchair trays. If babies are younger than six months, help them develop visual convergence (two eyes working together) by moving a dried color wheel in front of them from side to side and then from up to down. This activity will strengthen their tracking skills.

Toddlers
Toddlers will likely approach this project with enthusiasm! If they fill up their entire page with finger-paint art, take a pencil and draw some shapes on the wet paint. Tell them what you are drawing: "Here's a circle. Now, I'll draw a square." Toddlers may want to try tracing the shapes with their fingers. This is a great way to practice their drawing skills.

Preschoolers

Preschoolers may enjoy creating patterns with the finger paints. They can create a row of green thumbprints, then a row of blue thumbprints, and so on. Let them take the lead when creating this artwork.

School-Age Children

Have school-age children create bugs with their finger paints. To create a ladybug, they can use their thumbs to press red paint onto the paper and then make purple dots using their index fingers. To create a green caterpillar, they can make a line of green dots.

At first my toddler playmates did not like the feel of the squishy paint on their hands. I guess it was a texture thing. The good news is, it didn't take long for finger painting to become an all-time favorite art exploration.

—Lisa

A Village to Call Our Own

This village of recycled milk cartons is fun to create, design, and play with.

What You'll Need	All Ages	Babies	Toddlers	Preschoolers	School-Age Children
Empty milk cartons and small rocks	🖐				
Masking tape	🖐				
Construction paper	🖐				
Stickers			🖐	🖐	🖐
Child-safe scissors	🖐				
Markers			🖐	🖐	🖐
Glue stick			🖐	🖐	🖐
Picture of a building					🖐

Wash out empty milk cartons, then cut off the top of each. Place a small rock inside each carton to keep it steady. Using masking tape, cover the cartons with construction paper with the older playmates' help. Then the children can decorate their carton buildings with stickers, paper cutouts, or markers to create windows, doors, and other features. When the carton buildings are finished, the resulting village may include a home, a school, or other favorite places.

Babies

While older children are busy with their cartons, decorate one for each baby using brightly colored cutouts like a red circle, blue triangle, and yellow square. Place the cartons in front of

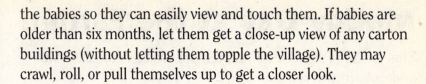

the babies so they can easily view and touch them. If babies are older than six months, let them get a close-up view of any carton buildings (without letting them topple the village). They may crawl, roll, or pull themselves up to get a closer look.

Toddlers

Give toddlers milk cartons that are already wrapped with construction paper. They will have fun decorating their structures with stickers. You can also give them a few paper shape cutouts to glue onto their structures. Name the shapes as you assist them with the glue.

Preschoolers

To help preschoolers make their buildings, have them lay the cartons on their sides on sheets of construction paper and use large pieces of masking tape to tape the paper to the cartons. Let them use their imaginations to create a haunted house, a castle, a library, or whatever they desire. Ask them what their building should look like: "Does it need a door? Some windows?"

School-Age Children

School-age children may want to design their own buildings or work from a picture of a building they wish to re-create. Images will serve as guides for window placement, exterior color, and so on.

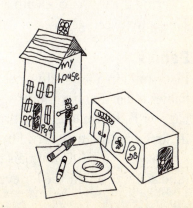

Muddy Day at the Farm

Kids can add edible "mud" to their art projects to create the perfect barnyard scenes!

What You'll Need	All Ages	Babies	Toddlers	Preschoolers	School-Age Children
Prepared chocolate pudding	🖐				
Plastic containers			🖐	🖐	🖐
Plastic tablecloth or newspaper			🖐	🖐	🖐
Large zip-close plastic bags		🖐			
Farm animal stickers			🖐		🖐
Construction paper			🖐	🖐	🖐
Crayons				🖐	🖐

Give small plastic containers of "mud" (chocolate pudding) to toddlers, preschoolers, and school-age children. We recommend covering the workspace with a plastic tablecloth or newspaper. This activity can get messy!

Babies

Place mud in a large zip-close plastic bag for each baby. For babies older than six months, let them squeeze the squishy bags with their hands for a great sensory experience. Be sure to supervise them closely. For babies younger than six months, sing a song to salute animals that love to roll around in mud (and squeeze a new toe for every "little piggy"):

This little piggy went to market.
This little piggy stayed home.
This little piggy ate roast beef.
This little piggy had none.
This little piggy went, "Wee, wee, wee," all the way home.

Toddlers
Most toddlers love to get messy, and this activity gives toddlers the perfect chance to do so. Have toddlers place some animal stickers on their construction paper and then use their hands to cover the stickers with chocolate mud!

Preschoolers
We know pigs love mud—show preschoolers how to draw a pig using shapes: Have them draw one large circle for the head and a smaller circle in the center for the snout. Then have them make small circle eyes and triangles on top of the large circle for ears. They can then cover their pigs with mud!

School-Age Children
School-age children may enjoy designing a barn on their paper before adding the animal stickers and the mud. Let them get creative with the mud by making a muddy swamp, a muddy trail, or a mud pile.

Icy Shapes

To keep your playmates entertained on a cold day or cool on a hot one, make ice that they can build with!

What You'll Need	All Ages	Babies	Toddlers	Preschoolers	School-Age Children
Plastic containers in various shapes and sizes (pie pans, ice cube trays, bowls, etc.)	✋				
Food coloring	✋				
Small toys or cereal			✋	✋	✋
Baking sheets			✋	✋	✋
Sponges				✋	✋

Fill the containers with water and add a few drops of food coloring to each. If you like, drop small toys (for older children) or cereal (for toddlers) in the water. Freeze the containers overnight. The next day, pop the shapes out of the containers and onto baking sheets. Then let the fun begin! What can the children build? Is it hard to hold the ice? How does it feel?

Babies

Babies older than six months can play with a piece of ice on their highchair trays. Make sure the ice is small enough for them to handle but large enough that they can't put it in their mouths. Also make sure it's not a piece with a toy or some cereal in it. As they try to reach for the ice, it may slip away. If they do grab it, how quickly do they sense the cold? Watch

closely as the ice melts, and take it away when it's small
enough to put in their mouths. If the babies are younger than
six months, run the ice along their toes for a second several
times. Baby feet have thousands of nerve endings, giving them
some "cool" sensations!

Toddlers
Toddlers may enjoy stacking ice cubes or sliding them up and
down the baking sheet as they begin to melt. They may be less
disappointed when the ice melts if you give them a piece with
a cereal surprise inside!

Preschoolers
Preschoolers will enjoy building with the ice pieces. To make
the frozen shapes stick together, tell preschoolers to use a
sponge to dab water onto the ice, then hold the pieces together
until they are firmly attached.

School-Age Children
School-age children may want to build with the ice, or they
may turn it into a hands-on learning experiment. Make some
predictions with them. How long will each shape take to melt?
Heat will melt them—what else will? Let them take a piece of
ice to the sink and run cold and warm water over it. Write
down their predictions and see how close they are to the
answers.

Host Tip

To make the ice sculptures last longer, freeze the baking sheets overnight as well. And for an easy way to get the ice out of the container, set the container in warm water for a few minutes, then the ice will slip out.

My preschool son loved this activity. He spent a lot of time seeing how he could get the ice to melt. He tried salt, pepper, and sugar and was pleased with his results!

—Heather

Marvelous Marble Roll

With this art project, kids will wiggle and move to make a marble create fabulous designs!

What You'll Need	All Ages	Babies	Toddlers	Preschoolers	School-Age Children
Plastic container with cover			🖐		
Shoebox with lid				🖐	
Larger cardboard box					🖐
Blanket	🖐				
Paper	🖐				
Washable tempera paint	🖐				
Marbles (or small balls)	🖐				
Wet wipes		🖐			
Tennis ball					🖐

Find a few containers for the children, like a clear plastic container with a cover for toddlers, a shoebox with a lid for preschoolers, and a large cardboard box for school-age children. (Or you can can keep this activity simple by having all children use similar containers.) Place a sheet of paper on the bottom of each container. Add a few dabs of paint to the paper, then drop a marble in each container. Children can shake and dip their containers from side to side so their marbles roll and make cool designs.

Babies

Lay babies on a blanket and get them ready to make a special marble design. Dab some paint on a marble and gently roll the marble around the sole of their feet, making any design you choose. They will find the sensation on their feet exhilarating. Press their feet onto paper, and their artwork is complete. Have wet wipes on hand so you can clean their feet as soon as the activity is done.

Toddlers

Teach toddlers what happens when they combine two colors in their containers. Place a dab of red paint and a dab of blue on the paper, put the marble in their container, and secure the cover. Encourage them to roll the marble around for a few minutes. When they open the container, what color do they see? It should resemble purple. You can also try combining red and yellow to make orange and blue and yellow to make green.

Preschoolers

Preschoolers may enjoy leaving off the shoebox's lid and trying to direct the marble across the paper as they dip the box from side to side. Or they may want to put the lid on so the marble's designs will be a surprise when they're finished.

School-Age Children

School-age children should work as a team (with each other or with you). One can hold one end of a larger box while the other holds the other end. Then work together to dip the box from side to side. Make a fun game by not letting the marble touch the sides of the box! If you like, try this game with a tennis ball instead of a marble.

Fruity Tie-Dye Shirts

Kids can create one-of-a-kind T-shirts using this centuries-old craft. Have the kids all wear their creations the next time they all get together!

What You'll Need	All Ages	Babies	Toddlers	Preschoolers	School-Age Children
Plain light-colored cotton T-shirts and/or onesies	🖐				
Rubber bands or string	🖐				
Fabric makers		🖐			
Spray bottle filled with water	🖐				
Large plastic trash bags	🖐				
Large pot	🖐				
Package of fruit drink mix (like Kool-Aid)	🖐				
Spoon	🖐				
Tongs	🖐				
Iron	🖐				

Babies

Using T-shirts, make buddies for the babies. Wrap some rubber bands lengthwise around a crumpled T-shirt to create a caterpillar. Use fabric markers to make eyes and smiling mouths. While the other children work with their T-shirts, start at the babies' feet and wiggle the caterpillar slowly up their bodies while singing this song:

The itsy-bitsy caterpillar crawled up the baby's leg,
(Crawl the caterpillar up the baby's leg.)
Wiggled the baby's tummy,
(Touch the tummy with the caterpillar.)
And jumped up to her head.
(Place the caterpillar on the baby's head.)
Down came a bug and kissed her on the face.
(Kiss baby with the caterpillar.)
And the itsy-bitsy caterpillar left without a trace.
(Hide the caterpillar behind your back.)

Toddlers, Preschoolers, and School-Age Children

Have toddlers, preschoolers, and school-age children dunk their T-shirts—plus one onesie for each baby—in a tub of water or spray them with a spray bottle. Make sure the shirts are completely wet. Lay a plastic bag on the ground for each child to serve as their work space. Have children crumple, fold, and twist the shirts to make them as small as possible (toddlers may need assistance). Then work together to bind the shirts tightly with rubber bands or string. To create the dye, make the fruit drink in a large pot. For four shirts, make four servings. For two shirts, make two servings. Kids can help stir.

While the kids watch from a safe distance, boil the fruit drink, then cool it to room temperature. Place the shirts in the mixture and let them soak for twenty minutes. To make the wait go faster for the kids, ask them to predict what the shirts will look like when they're done or have them sing the "Itsy-Bitsy Caterpillar" song to the baby. You could also play a few activities from the Out & About Chapter, like Freeze! (page 168) and Ten Things (page 180).

After the shirts have soaked, remove them from the pot using tongs. The children will enjoy their fruity scent. Pull a chair up to the sink so older kids can take turns watching you run cold water over each shirt, or do this step outside with the hose. The kids can tell you when the water runs clear. Remove the rubber bands and rinse the shirts again. Kids can help hang the shirts to dry. Iron them if necessary once dry, then wear them!

Colorful Collages

Enjoy some colorful drawings by creating a collage of images.

What You'll Need	All Ages	Babies	Toddlers	Preschoolers	School-Age Children
Crayons			🖐	🖐	🖐
Coloring books			🖐	🖐	🖐
White construction paper			🖐		
Colorful blankets or pillow cases		🖐			
Towels					
Child-safe scissors			🖐	🖐	🖐
Construction paper in various colors			🖐		
Glue sticks			🖐	🖐	🖐
Poster board				🖐	

To begin this activity, preschoolers and school-age children can color some pages from favorite coloring books, and toddlers can color on white construction paper. They'll then use these colorful images to design collages.

Babies

While older children work on their collages, you can create a blanket collage for babies to explore. Layer and angle three to four different-colored blankets or pillow cases on the floor. Make a bolster by rolling a few towels together lengthwise, then place the babies on their tummies over the bolster so they have a great view of the collage. Looking at colorful patterns will help a baby's brain and vision develop. Babies are particularly interested in bright colors.

Toddlers

Cut out several shapes from the white construction paper the toddlers colored, as well as from other sheets of construction paper. Ask them to identify the shapes and colors. With your help, toddlers can glue the shapes onto a sheet of construction paper.

Preschoolers

At this age, many preschoolers can begin to use a pair of child-safe scissors. This activity is a great way to help preschoolers develop this skill. Tear out the pages they have colored from their coloring books. Make sure they feature fairly large images for them to cut out. Then they can glue the images onto poster board.

School-Age Children

When school-age children finish cutting out images from the coloring books, encourage them to arrange the drawings in a fun pattern—upside down or even overlapping—before they glue the images in place. They may even want to use crayons to create a backdrop or scene for their collages.

We glued some of the collages made into an old note-book. The kids love to leaf through them from time to time!

—Lisa

King and Queen Crowns

Who wouldn't enjoy being king or queen for the day? Everyone can enjoy the prestige that comes with these easy-to-make crowns!

What You'll Need	All Ages	Babies	Toddlers	Preschoolers	School-Age Children
Child-safe scissors	🖐				
Construction paper in various colors	🖐				
Art supplies, such as crayons, stickers, stamps, cotton balls, aluminum foil, and so on	🖐				
Tape	🖐				
Glue	🖐				
Paper plate		🖐			🖐
Glitter					🖐

For each crown, cut a sheet of construction paper into two strips lengthwise—one strip two inches wide and the other about six inches wide. Let children decorate the six-inch strips with a variety of art supplies. When they've finished, tape the two strips together in a circle, adjusting the narrower strip to fit the circumference of each child's head.

Babies

While older children create their crowns, you can introduce babies to different textures. Simply glue a few of the crown materials (such a cotton ball, foil, and some tape) to a paper plate. Place babies' hands on each item and tell them what they are touching. Provide one-word descriptions such as "soft," "crunchy," and "smooth." Also, have their playmates make and decorate crowns for them. Perhaps school-age children can write a term of endearment on it such as "Our Little Prince!"

Toddlers

Toddlers can decorate their crowns with stickers, crayons, and stamps. To create jewels, cut diamond shapes from construction paper and help toddlers glue them onto their crowns. They can also add cotton balls or pieces of foil to their dazzling headpieces. Write their names on their crowns.

Preschoolers

Preschoolers may want to cut their own construction paper strips for their crowns, which is a great opportunity to work on their scissor skills. To help them, fold their construction paper at the two-inch mark and let them follow the crease with their scissors. If they desire, they can cut patterns along the top of the six-inch strip to add designs to their crown.

School-Age Children

School-age children's crowns can sparkle with a bit of glitter. Have them put glue on their crowns and sprinkle glitter over the glue. Have them tip the crowns and gently tap the excess glitter onto paper plates. Allow the glue to dry.

Host Tip

To get into the spirit, address the children as "King" or "Queen" when they wear their crowns. This is a great photo opportunity!

> My son and daughter wore their crowns the entire day. They even made one for me to wear!
>
> —Heather

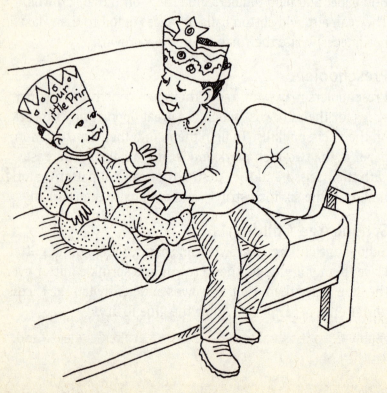

Goobly-Goop

This fun, goopy substance changes from solid to liquid with a touch of your hand.

What You'll Need	All Ages	Babies	Toddlers	Preschoolers	School-Age Children
½ cup cornstarch	🖐				
¼ cup water	🖐				
Food coloring	🖐				
Pie pans	🖐				
Zip-close plastic bags		🖐			
Plastic spoon and cups			🖐		
Small plastic toys				🖐	
Seashell or rock collection				🖐	

To make goobly-goop, mix the cornstarch, water, and food coloring in a pie pan for each child. Older children may want to help, especially with the food coloring. The finished substance will thrill the children: Upon first touch, it feels solid, but it quickly turns to liquid when tiny fingers touch it, generating heat.

Babies

If babies are younger than six months, lay them on their backs and let them kick a clean pie pan with their feet while older playmates play with the goop. They'll like metallic bangs they can create. If babies are older, place their portions of the goobly-goop in zip-close plastic bags. Let them squeeze and pat the bags.

Toddlers

At the beginning of the activity, let toddlers decide what color they'd like you to make their goobly-goop. Once the substance is ready, toddlers can discover different ways to handle it using tools, such as a spoon and cups. For example, they may decide to transfer the goop from cup to cup with the spoon.

Preschoolers

As you prepare the goobly-goop, have preschoolers add their own food coloring to create the perfect shade. After exploring the goop with their hands, encourage them to play with small plastic toys in the goop. The goop can make toy car tracks disappear or, if thick enough, hold a figurine in place.

School-Age Children

To thicken the consistency, have school-age children add more cornstarch to their goop. Thicker goop will hold things in place and may be perfect for arranging a seashell or rock collection. They can also put some goop in their hands and drip it over a clean pan to write out their name or initials.

Canvas Painting

This activity uses a huge canvas to encourage free artistic expression that is full of possibilities!

What You'll Need	All Ages	Babies	Toddlers	Preschoolers	School-Age Children
Old flat sheet	✋				
Clothesline or 2 chairs, a rope, and 2 clothespins	✋				
Washable tempera paint	✋				
Sponges			✋		
Paintbrushes				✋	
Spray bottles					✋

The outdoors may be the best place for this activity, but you can do it indoors if you have enough room. If you're outdoors, hang an old sheet on a clothesline, making sure children can easily reach it. If you're indoors or if you don't have a clothesline, set up two chairs and tie a rope between them. Lay the sheet over the rope. Children will have a blast decorating the "canvas."

Babies

Before the painting begins, sit next to the hanging sheet with the babies. Older children may even engage in a game of peek-aboo with them! Have babies touch the sheet with their hands and their feet. To encourage artistic expression, put a little paint on their fingers and let them smear the sheet. Even though tempera paint is nontoxic, supervise babies closely so they don't put their fingers in their mouths.

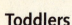

Toddlers
Toddlers will enjoy decorating the canvas using sponges dipped in paint. They can blot or smear paint onto the sheet.

Preschoolers
This activity will challenge preschoolers' motor skills. Encourage them to paint the top part of the canvas with paintbrushes; they'll need to reach above chest level and use the muscles required to write—a great exercise for the future!

School-Age Children
Fill spray bottles half with paint and half with water. School-age children can squirt the sheet to create unique designs.

Host Tip
Use the finished painting to decorate a playroom or other space in your home.

Stay-Still Art

We know kids don't usually stay still for long, but this still-life art project will inspire them to stay at rest!

What You'll Need	All Ages	Babies	Toddlers	Preschoolers	School-Age Children
Still-life art (see suggestions below)	🖐				
Drawing paper			🖐	🖐	🖐
Crayons			🖐	🖐	🖐
Pencils					🖐

Make a still-life art setting on the center of the kitchen table. You can use stuffed animals, a bowl of fruit, a vase with flowers, some colorful mugs, or any household decoration. Hand out paper and crayons and encourage the older children to draw what they see. There is no right or wrong in art, as long as making it is fun!

Babies

Young babies can see bold, contrasting colors, but it will be a while before they can identify the names of each. In the meantime, introduce the babies to colors through touch, using objects from the still-life art setting. For example, rub a flower petal on a baby's cheek and say, "This purple petal is smooth." Gently dip a baby's hand in a glass of cool water and say, "This clear water is cool." Snuggle a teddy bear on a baby's chest and say, "This brown bear is soft."

Toddlers

Help toddlers study the still-life setting. They may be particularly interested if it includes objects with which they are familiar, like favorite stuffed animals. What colors and shapes do they see? They may be able to match colors they see with the crayons for their drawings.

Preschoolers

This activity should be a fun exercise for preschoolers. As they enter the preschool years, their drawings may become more defined with specific shapes and colors. To help them get started, they may prefer that you draw an outline of the setting they can trace over with their crayons. Teach them how to make dark marks by firmly pressing their crayons and light ones by brushing the crayons softly over the paper.

School-Age Children

Encourage school-age children to take their time studying the objects placed on the table. They can study shapes, light contrasts, and textures. Suggest they sketch the setting first using a pencil. Once they are satisfied with the sketches, they can color in the objects.

Surprise Designs

Kids will love to see their colorful designs magically reappear in this activity.

What You'll Need	All Ages	Babies	Toddlers	Preschoolers	School-Age Children
White construction paper	✋				
Crayons	✋				
Scissors		✋			
Paintbrushes			✋	✋	✋
Diluted black tempera paint			✋	✋	✋
Clear plastic water bottles and small colored objects		✋			
Rubber bands			✋		
White chalk					✋

Give older children sheets of white construction paper. Encourage them to draw, scribble, and color the entire sheet with crayons. Cut a one-inch-wide strip from each of their papers for the babies' part of the activity. After cutting the strips, have children paint diluted black paint all over their papers. As the paint dries, their designs will reveal themselves. The paint is water based and thus less dense than the crayon markings, allowing the colors to pop through!

Babies

Place the one-inch strips into a clear plastic water bottle for each baby. Secure each bottle tightly, and let the babies explore the colors within. You also can create a red bottle, a blue bottle, and a green bottle by placing objects of corresponding colors inside each. For instance, place an appropriately colored, peeled crayon in each bottle. Ask older children to find other appropriately colored objects to add. Preschoolers may add a piece of blue construction paper to the blue bottle or a piece of red apple skin to the red bottle.

Toddlers

Use a rubber band to wrap three crayons together. Toddlers' small hands will have an easier time holding them, and they'll be able to add many colors to their papers instantly. When it's time to add the black paint, they may also appreciate larger paintbrushes that will let them paint broader strokes.

Preschoolers

For fun, write preschoolers' names in large bubble letters across their papers. Have them color in the letters with squiggly lines, stripes, or crisscrossed lines. They'll enjoy seeing their names appear when the paint dries.

School-Age Children

Suggest that school-age children create mazes with crayons. They can start with large squares with an entrance and exit. Then they can create mazes of tunnels to connect the entrance and exit. Have them add some blocked areas as well. Once the paint dries, they can use white chalk to complete the maze.

> My son drew a rainbow. He loved watching the colors reappear.
>
> —Heather

Apple Art

We know apples are good to eat, but they're also good for creating deliciously fun art.

What You'll Need	All Ages	Babies	Toddlers	Preschoolers	School-Age Children
Apples (any variety)	✋				
Knife	✋				
Popsicle sticks			✋	✋	✋
Washable tempera paint			✋	✋	✋
Paper plates			✋	✋	✋
Sheets of white paper			✋	✋	✋
Yogurt		✋			
Butcher paper				✋	✋
Crayons				✋	✋

Cut the apples vertically in half. With the flat side down, vertically insert a Popsicle stick into the center of the apple. Each child can use these homemade "stamps" to make a painting. Pour paint onto paper plates, then have the children dip the apples into the paint and gently press them onto paper.

Babies

Take each baby's hand and explore an apple half together. Let them smell and touch the fruit. If babies are over six months and eating dairy, you can place some yogurt on their highchair tray as edible "paint." Closely supervise them as they swirl the apple around in the yogurt.

Toddlers

Show toddlers how to use the stamp by holding the stick, pressing the apple onto the paper, and then lifting it up. Or instead of stamping the page, they may choose to use the apple as a paintbrush. Let them do so!

Preschoolers and School-Age Children

Preschoolers and school-age children can create their own apple tree painting. Lay a large sheet of butcher paper on the floor and encourage them to use crayons to draw a tree outline, including branches and leaves. Then they can add apples to the tree by using their apple stamps. How many apples can their tree hold?

Host Tip

When you're done creating apple art, teach preschoolers and school-age children how to begin the process of planting an apple tree. Children can put their seeds in a paper towel, place them in their home refrigerator, and keep their paper towel moist for a week or so. When they notice sprouts, it is time to transfer the sprouts to a cup with soil. Place the cup on a sunny windowsill and keep the soil moist. In a week, the sprouts will be ready to be planted outside. Choose a sunny location and continue to water them. With love and care, you will have more apples to eat and use for art! You may even want to plant two sprouts because apple trees grow best in pairs.

Pipe Cleaner Flowers

Children can bend and twist pipe cleaners to create flowers that will brighten any room!

What You'll Need	All Ages	Babies	Toddlers	Preschoolers	School-Age Children
Small bells		🖐			
Pipe cleaners	🖐				
Glue	🖐				
Construction paper		🖐	🖐		
Paintbrushes			🖐	🖐	🖐
Washable tempera paint	🖐				
Wax paper				🖐	🖐
String				🖐	🖐

Babies

Attach a small bell to a pipe cleaner and gently secure it to each baby's ankle. Each time they kick, crawl, or move their legs, they will hear the bells jingle. They'll love the gentle sound and the soft feel of the pipe cleaner against their skin. For the babies' flowers, make circles with green pipe cleaners and glue them onto construction paper. Once the glue dries, you can dip their index fingers into yellow paint and gently press it around the green circle to create petals.

Toddlers

Most toddlers will enjoy the fuzzy feel and flexibility of pipe cleaners. Let toddlers play with their pipe cleaners, bending them into whatever design they choose. Give them several to twist together, and help them glue them onto construction paper. They can use paint to create pretty flowers to embellish their pipe cleaner designs.

Preschoolers and School-Age Children

Show preschoolers and school-age children how to create a flower made from pipe cleaners. (Most preschoolers will be able to create the circles but may need assistance with other steps.)

- Leaves: Bend a pipe cleaner into a circle and twist it closed. Then twist the circle in the center, creating a figure eight. Mold into leaf shapes.

- Petals: Bend a pipe cleaner into a circle and twist it closed. Then twist the circle in the center, creating a figure eight. Mold into petal shapes. Repeat with another pipe cleaner. Twist the four petals together to create a bloom shape.

- Stem: Attach the leaves in the middle of a pipe cleaner and twist the flower to the top.

Lay the design on wax paper and squeeze glue into the empty spaces of the petals. When it is dry, children can fill in the petals with paint. Then help them cut away the excess wax paper, tie string to the pipe cleaner flowers, and hang them by a window.

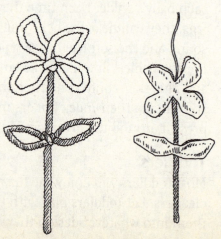

Spin, Spin Pinwheel

This spinning wheel of color will dazzle children.

What You'll Need	All Ages	Babies	Toddlers	Preschoolers	School-Age Children
Scissors	🖐				
Ledger-size printing paper	🖐				
Crayons	🖐				
Stickers	🖐				
Pencil	🖐				
Pin	🖐				
Dowel	🖐				

Note: The materials above will create one pinwheel, but you may decide to have older children each make their own with your assistance. For each pinwheel, cut ledger paper into a large square. Put it within everyone's reach on a table. Have children decorate the front and back with crayons and stickers. School-age children may want to write the names of each playmate on it. Let older children assist with the assembly:

1. Fold the paper from opposite corner to opposite corner, and then unfold. Do the same for the other corners.
2. Make a pencil mark on each fold about one-third of the distance from the center.
3. Cut along the folds, stopping at the pencil marks. This will create eight points.
4. Fold every other point to the center.
5. Stick a pin through all four points. The head of the pin will

form the hub of the pinwheel.
6. Stick the pin into a thin dowel.
7. Enjoy!

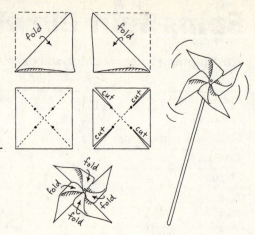

Babies

Babies love to watch colorful, moving objects. Sit with them as you gently blow on the pinwheel and let them enjoy the visual display.

Toddlers

Teach toddlers how to move the pinwheel by making an O shape with their lips and blowing onto the center of the pinwheel.

Preschoolers and School-Age Children

Preschoolers and school-age children may decide to create their own pinwheels with different themes. Before pinning their pinwheels together, they can use crayons to create a patriotic, springtime, or rainbow theme.

Did You Know?

On the annual International Day of Peace (September 21), people should plant pinwheels outdoors as a public statement of peace. The spinning pinwheels represent the peaceful thoughts and feelings spinning throughout the world!

Faces Fit for a Frame

Use empty CD cases to create easy-to-display picture frames.

What You'll Need	All Ages	Babies	Toddlers	Preschoolers	School-Age Children
Empty CD cases	🖐				
Child-safe scissors	🖐				
Construction paper	🖐				
Photos of all the children (or photocopies of photos)	🖐				
Crayons, stickers, or puzzle pieces	🖐				
Tape or glue stick	🖐				
Pencils			🖐		🖐

For each case, cut two pieces of construction paper: one to cover the case's inside front cover, and another to cover the CD tray. Help children select photos of their faces to glue onto one of the pieces, then they can decorate around the photo with crayons or stickers. They'll decorate the second piece of paper according to their age-specific instructions below. When both pieces are finished, use tape or glue to affix one to the inside front cover and the other over the tray.

Babies

Flip through photos with the babies while the other children work on their projects. Babies love to study friendly faces. Tell them who is in each photo. You or older children can also create a frame for each baby. Place some photos of the baby with her playmates in the frame as a great keepsake of this activity.

Toddlers

Give toddlers some stickers or puzzle pieces to decorate around their photos. (Help them with the glue.) You can also use a pencil to record recent milestones on the other piece of paper. Remember to include the date.

Preschoolers

At this age, some preschoolers can draw faces with appropriate features. Have preschoolers choose a photo to glue onto one side of the case, then have them draw a picture of the photo on the second piece. They'll use their developing observational and drawing skills to duplicate features.

School-Age Children

On the second piece of paper, school-age children can write a narrative about what is happening in the photo they glued onto the other piece. What are they doing in the photo? How are they feeling?

Host Tip
This activity makes great gifts for friends and relatives!

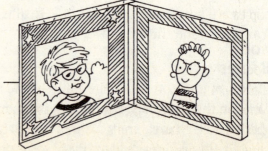

Wild Animal Flashcards

Create your very own flashcards using animal images from magazines and coloring books.

What You'll Need	All Ages	Babies	Toddlers	Preschoolers	School-Age Children
Old magazines or coloring books	🖐				
Child-safe scissors			🖐	🖐	🖐
Glue stick			🖐	🖐	🖐
Large index cards			🖐	🖐	🖐
Colored pencils or markers					🖐

You or older children can begin this activity by finding animal images in magazines or coloring books. They can then cut out and glue the images onto index cards.

Babies
Babies will love the ripping, tearing, and crinkling of the pages in glossy magazines. They'll enjoy seeing the contrasting, bright images and hearing the pages rip. If they like, older children can flip through the magazines and describe the images to the babies.

Toddlers
Toddlers will enjoy finding animal images for their flashcards. This task will help develop their ability to classify objects. Once they find animals, be sure to ask them, "What animal is this?" and, "What sound does this animal make?" Help them glue the images onto index cards.

Preschoolers

Challenge preschoolers to sort their animal images according to size, habitation (land or sea), and other groupings before gluing them onto the index cards. This is a great way to sharpen their organizational and observational skills. Be sure to ask them, "Which group do you have the most of?" or, "What is your favorite animal and why?"

School-Age Children

Encourage school-age children to strengthen their drawing skills by making symmetry art. Have them cut an animal image in half and glue one half onto an index card. Challenge them to draw the other half of the image, using colored pencils or markers.

Recyclables

With imagination, children can create cars, figurines, or their own inventions using recyclable materials.

What You'll Need	All Ages	Baby	Toddler	Preschooler	School-Age Child
Recyclable materials (including empty toilet paper or paper towel rolls, egg cartons, aluminum foil, Popsicle sticks, plastic cups, tissue paper, and so on)	✋				
Grocery bags			✋	✋	✋
Art supplies (including crayons, construction paper, masking tape, wax paper, pipe cleaners, and pompoms)			✋	✋	✋
Contact paper		✋			✋

Place various recyclable items into separate grocery bags for toddlers, preschoolers, and school-age children. As children pull out the objects, they'll be busy imagining the different ways they can use each object. Also provide them with art supplies to help them turn the recyclables into whatever their imagination desires. This activity requires lots of artistic expression and creativity.

Babies

Tape a small piece of contact paper sticky side up in front of each baby. Slowly stick an empty toilet paper roll to the paper, then peel it off. If babies are six months or older, encourage them to stick and peel off the roll themselves. By eight months, most babies can solve simple problems like getting an object by pulling it. No matter their age, they'll enjoy the tearing sound.

Toddlers

Toddlers will love to sort and explore the objects in their bags. If possible, make sure to put an egg carton in each one. They'll love this wonderful organizer. For example, they can use it to sort pompoms according to color. Or they may choose to use the cartons for different activities. For example: Flip the egg carton over and poke Popsicle sticks through the bottom of each cup. Children will have fun moving them in and out.

Preschoolers

Preschoolers will enjoy finding new uses for the recyclables, such as making their own pencil holders from a large plastic cup and some masking tape. Have them use small strips of masking tape to completely cover the cup in layered designs.

School-Age Children

School-age children may decide to create three-dimensional scenes by sticking their objects to contact paper. Ideas include a playground (they can cut a toilet paper roll in half lengthwise to create a slide or use Popsicle sticks to create monkey bars) or a garden (they can make a colorful flower patch with colored tissue paper). A decorated sheet of construction paper can serve as the backdrop to any scene. Simply have them make a stiff crease one inch from one side of the construction paper and attach the fold to the contact paper.

My son loved making inventions with recyclable materials. The most memorable one was a "candy maker." He explained to me in detail how the contraption works, and he worked on it for over an hour!

—Heather

Let Our Feet Do the Painting

Children will love using their feet to create art in this activity.

What You'll Need	All Ages	Babies	Toddlers	Preschoolers	School-Age Children
Newspapers and/or old shower curtain	🖐				
Tape	🖐				
Sheets of plain art paper	🖐				
Washable tempera paint	🖐				
2–4 large, flat pans	🖐				
Medium-size paintbrushes	🖐				
Wet wipes	🖐				
Toy cars or plastic dinosaurs				🖐	
Crayons					🖐

Ask the children to dress in old clothes; shorts may be best. Spread newspapers or an old shower curtain on the floor, then tape enough plain art paper on top to create a four-by-eight-foot walking space for each child. Pour paint into two large, flat pans and then have kids remove their shoes and socks. Before you paint their feet, make sure the children know they must stay on the art paper and newspaper until you clean their feet with wet wipes at the end of the project!

Babies

Babies will enjoy the sensation of the cool, wet paint on the soles of their tiny feet. If babies are younger than six months, have them sit on an adult's lap as they kneel next to the paper. Gently press their painted feet onto the paper. If babies are older than six months, help them "walk" across the paper. This activity is a perfect way to capture some of their first steps.

Toddlers

Toddlers may want to help paint the soles of their playmates' feet. They'll love to have their feet painted, too, and they'll enjoy walking across the paper. Encourage them to tiptoe, slide, or stomp.

Preschoolers

Encourage preschoolers to create dance patterns or other creative designs with their feet. To make some crazy tracks, they can dip their toy cars' wheels or plastic dinosaurs' feet into the paint and roll or walk them across the paper. They may want to even design a map.

School-Age Children

School-age children can use crayons to draw a hopscotch grid on their paper before painting their feet. Ten numbered squares in a column make up a traditional hopscotch grid: Start with three single squares in a column, follow them with two squares side by side, then one single, then two squares side by side, and finally two single ones. After painting their feet, they can hop through a game. When the paint dries, they'll have a fun hopscotch practice mat to use with their friends.

I make sure the kids wear play clothes for this activity. My niece wanted to examine the paint on her feet and lost her balance, making a very cute "bum" print on the paper!

—Lisa

Did You Know?
There are over seventy-five thousand nerve endings in your feet. This activity stimulates these nerves, creating a heightened state of awareness in children.

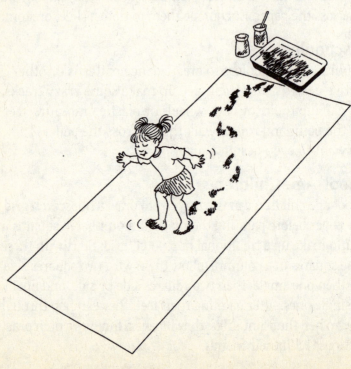

Very Cool Fruity Play Dough

This play dough has a yummy and fruity scent! Plus, it's safe to taste!

What You'll Need	All Ages	Babies	Toddlers	Preschoolers	School-age children
Homemade play dough (see recipe below)	🖐				
Wax paper	🖐				
Kitchen gadgets (including a potato masher, spatula, rolling pin, plastic cookie cutters, and plastic knife)				🖐	🖐
Child-safe scissors				🖐	🖐
Tree leaves				🖐	🖐

Play Dough Recipe
½ cup salt
2 cups water
Fruit drink mix (like Kool-Aid)
2 tablespoons vegetable oil
2 cups sifted flour
2 tablespoons alum

Combine salt and water in saucepan and boil until the salt dissolves. Remove from heat and tint with fruit drink mix. Add oil, flour, and alum. Knead until smooth. This dough will last two months in an airtight container or zip-close freezer bag.

Preschoolers and school-age children can help you prepare the play dough. When it has cooled, they can divide it evenly

339

among their friends. The children will love the fun, fruity scent. Have children line their workspaces with wax paper.

Babies

If babies are younger than six months, hold some play dough close to their noses so they can smell the fruity aroma. If they're older, let them explore a small amount under your supervision. Together, form the dough into the shape of a cake while singing:

> *Patty-cake, patty-cake, baker's man.*
> *Bake me a cake as fast as you can.*
> *Roll it, pat it, mark it with a* B,
> *and put it in the oven for baby and me.*

Toddlers

Toddlers may choose to bang, pound, and roll their play dough into various shapes and sizes. Show them how to flatten the dough and press their hands in it to create handprints.

Preschoolers and School-Age Children

Here are some ways preschoolers and school-age children can have fun with their play dough:

- Make cookies: Use kitchen gadgets to roll out the dough and cut out cookie shapes.
- Practice using scissors: This dough slices easily and grips the child-safe scissors better than paper does.
- Create leaf imprints: Flatten the dough and press leaves into it.
- Make figurines: Design clowns, cars, and other objects.

Four Seasons

Celebrate the four seasons by finger-painting pictures representing the special things that happen each season.

What You'll Need	All Ages	Babies	Toddlers	Preschoolers	School-Age Children
Construction paper	🖐				
Marker	🖐				
Washable tempera paint	🖐				
Wet wipes	🖐				

Label four sheets of construction paper, each with a different season: "Winter," "Spring," "Summer," and "Fall." Below you'll find examples of paintings the children can make with paint and their hands. (Have wet wipes close by for cleanup.) We've assigned an age group to each season, but the activities are easily interchangeable.

Winter
Babies can create a snowman to depict this cold season. Close their fists and dip them into blue paint. Press their hands onto the paper three times to create the three stacked balls of a snowman. For snowflakes, dip their fingers in white paint and dot the paint all over. When the paint is dry, you can draw a face and arms on the snowman.

Spring

Create a garden scene with toddlers. To make each flower, paint their hands with whatever color they each want, press down their hands to create the blooms, and then use green paint to make stems. Paint their other hand a different color to add more flowers. Another option is to draw a butterfly outline and have them dip their fingers in paint to create bright patterns for the wings.

Summer

What do preschoolers associate with the summer months? They may decide to create a sun by painting their closed fist yellow and pressing it down on the paper. They may also want to create ocean waves by using blue paint and their fingers to make squiggly lines. They could even create Fourth of July fireworks using brightly colored finger dots with streak marks trailing down.

Fall

School-age children will likely associate this time of year with falling leaves. Cover their palms, fingers, and the underside of their forearms with brown paint. When they press their arms and hands on the paper, they will make a tree trunk and branches. They can cover their other fingers with fall-like colors to add some leaves on the branches and on the ground.

Chapter 10

In the Kitchen

"One of my favorite activities to do during playdates is to share a meal or snack together. It's a time to talk, share ideas, and get kids' bellies full before some more fun!"

—Heather

Busy playmates will eventually get hungry. The best part is that they will have fun and learn the importance of teamwork!

The recipes in this chapter provide tasty and easy things our children have enjoyed making with us. While the process of following the recipe was fun for our kids, they especially loved eating the product—no meal is quite so delicious as one kids help make!

Children of all ages can help prepare these recipes. After choosing a recipe, read it through with the children and explain any unknown words. Gather the necessary ingredients and supplies. In each recipe, we suggest specific ways toddlers, preschoolers, and school-age children can help, and below you'll find additional ideas for how your "assistant chefs" can help prepare any recipe with your supervision:

Babies
- Watch all the action from a highchair or bouncy seat.
- Smell the food as it cooks.

- Play with measuring cups or a clean, easy-to-hold food item like an apple or potato.
- "Supervise" fellow assistant chefs.

Toddlers
- Pour and mix premeasured dry ingredients.
- Spread butter, margarine, peanut butter, and other spreads.
- Roll dough into balls.
- Grease pans with fingers.

Preschoolers
- Wash fruits and vegetables.
- Measure dry ingredients.
- Arrange items on a baking sheet.
- Crack eggs.

School-Age Children
- Peel vegetables.
- Slice fruits and vegetables.
- Measure liquid ingredients.
- Use the mixer.

Although the kitchen is certainly an exciting environment, it's also a hazardous one for unsupervised children. Always keep dangerous objects out of children's reach and closely supervise children using sharp utensils or hot appliances. In fact, until you're certain of a child's abilities, make it a rule that only an adult can handle these items. Make sure to emphasize healthy

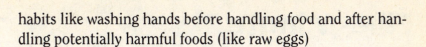

habits like washing hands before handling food and after handling potentially harmful foods (like raw eggs)

For more mealtime fun, check out "Packin' a Picnic" on page 19.

Five-Minute Scrambled Eggs

Early-day playdate plans? Kids will scramble to help make these delicious eggs!

4 eggs
4 tablespoons milk
4 tablespoons cottage cheese or shredded cheese
1 cup chopped green pepper, spinach, or other vegetable

1. Crack the eggs and pour the contents into a bowl. Preschoolers can do this task. Make sure they wash their hands thoroughly after handling the eggs.
2. Beat the eggs with a fork until the liquid is yellow.
3. Stir in the milk, cheese, and vegetables. School-age children can measure these ingredients and add them to the beaten eggs, and toddlers can help you stir the contents.
4. Spray a pan with cooking spray, then heat the pan over medium heat.
5. Cook the egg mixture, stirring occasionally until firm, about 5 minutes. This recipe makes 4 servings.

> My sisters and I loved making these eggs as kids. In fact, we coined the phrase "five-minute scrambled eggs" because we worked as a team and had our breakfast on the table in no time at all!
>
> —Heather

Mac & Cheese

This recipe is from Trish Kuffner's *The Children's Busy Book* (Meadowbrook Press), and it's one of our family's favorites! We've adapted it so all your kids can help prepare it.

2 cups uncooked macaroni
2 tablespoons butter
1 small onion, minced
   (optional)
1 tablespoon all-purpose flour

1 teaspoon salt
¼ teaspoon dry mustard
Dash of pepper
1½ cups milk
2 cups shredded Cheddar

1. Preheat oven to 350°F. Cook and drain the macaroni according to package instructions, then put it in a bowl. Set aside.
2. Toddlers can grease a 2-quart casserole dish. Unwrap one end of a stick of butter to rub all over the bottom and sides of the dish.
3. Melt 2 tablespoons butter in a saucepan over medium heat. If you like, add the onion and sauté it until tender.
4. Combine the flour, salt, mustard, and pepper in a small bowl. Preschoolers can do this task. Stir the mixture into the butter, then slowly stir in the milk.
5. Cook mixture, stirring constantly, until smooth and slightly thickened.
6. Remove the saucepan from heat. Add cheese, stir until melted.
7. Put the cooked macaroni in the casserole and pour the cheese mixture over the macaroni. School-age children can do this step.
8. Bake the macaroni until bubbly, about 20 minutes. This recipe makes 4 servings as a main dish or 6 servings as a side dish.

Taco Volcano

This twist on a Mexican favorite may encourage children to try new foods!

1 package large soft tortillas
1 pound lean ground beef
1 package taco seasoning
1 can refried beans
Sliced avocado
Mild salsa
Sour cream
Grated cheese

1. Cook the beef over medium-high heat until it's no longer pink. Drain the fat, then mix in the taco seasoning according to package instructions.
2. Place the beef, refried beans, avocado, salsa, sour cream, and cheese in individual bowls on the table.
3. Have children each lay a tortilla on a plate and spoon a small mound of refried beans onto it to make a mountain.
4. Children can then place avocado slices around the edge of the tortilla to make grass. They can spoon beef around the refried beans to create a rocky landscape around the mountain.
5. To turn the mountain into a volcano, the children can top the refried beans with salsa, sour cream, and cheese to create lava and ash.
6. To eat the taco volcano, roll it up and enjoy!

Pizza Faces

Personal-size pizzas get some personality with this fun recipe!

Pizza sauce
English muffins (one half per child)
Toppings, like bell pepper strips, olives and
   cherry tomatoes (cut in half), mushroom slices,
   ham slices, and pineapple pieces
Shredded cheese

1. Preheat your oven to 350°F.
2. Use a spoon to spread pizza sauce on half of an English muffin. Preschoolers and school-age children can do this step, and toddlers can do it with your help.
3. Arrange the toppings to make a face on the muffin. Encourage children to use toppings they don't regularly eat. Even picky eaters will want to eat their personal creations! Top with shredded cheese and place on a baking sheet.
4. Bake the pizzas for 10 minutes or until cheese is melted.

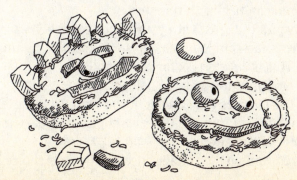

Fruity Pastry Cups

Kids will love to making these pastry cups as much as they'll love eating them!

Vegetable oil
9-inch refrigerated pie crust, thawed (We suggest
  Pillsbury Refrigerated Pie Crust.)
8-ounce tub of cottage cheese
Fruit toppings, such as strawberries, diced apples,
  pineapples, or bananas

1. Preheat your oven to 450°F.
2. Lightly grease a muffin pan with vegetable oil. This is a good task for a toddler: Put a few drops of oil in each muffin cup and let the child spread it with a pastry brush or a piece of paper towel.
3. Roll the pie crust out on a piece of wax paper. Press a plastic cup (about 5 inches in diameter) upside down onto the pie crust to cut circles. You should be able to make 8–10 circles. Children can help with this step.
4. Gently pull the crust with your hands to stretch each circle a bit. Press each circle into a cup so it resembles a muffin-cup liner. This is a good task for preschoolers.
5. Bake for 6 minutes or until golden.
6. After the pastries have cooled for at least 10 minutes, school-age children can fill each cup three-quarters full with cottage cheese.
7. Children can top the cottage cheese with their choice of fruit.

Oatmeal Pancakes

Here's another favorite from Trish Kuffner's *The Children's Busy Book* (Meadowbrook Press). We've adapted this recipe so kids can help make these pancakes with a twist.

½ cup all-purpose flour
½ cup quick-cooking oats
¾ cup buttermilk
¼ cup milk
1 tablespoon sugar
2 tablespoons vegetable oil

1 teaspoon baking powder
½ teaspoon baking soda
½ teaspoon salt
1 egg
Toppings, such as butter and
  syrup, applesauce, or jam

1. Pour all the ingredients except the toppings into a large bowl. Preschoolers can add the liquid ingredients, and toddlers can add the dry ingredients.
2. Beat the ingredients until the batter is smooth. Children can take turns doing this step.
3. For each pancake, pour ¼ cup of batter onto a hot nonstick griddle or frying pan. School-age children can help with this step.
4. Fry the pancakes until they bubble and their edges are dry. Flip the pancakes and cook the other sides until they're golden brown.
5. Serve the pancakes with butter and syrup, applesauce, or jam. This recipe makes 10–12 pancakes.

Host Tip
If you don't have buttermilk, substitute with 1 cup milk plus 1¾ tablespoons cream of tartar.

Tasty Banana Bread

This banana bread is a healthy afternoon snack or bedtime treat.

4 ripe bananas
⅓ cup butter, melted
¾–1 cup sugar
1 egg, beaten

1 teaspoon vanilla
1 teaspoon baking soda
Pinch of salt
1½ cups all-purpose flour

1. Preheat your oven to 350°F.
2. A toddler can grease a 4-by-8-inch loaf pan. Unwrap one end of a stick of butter and have the toddler rub it all over the bottom and sides of the pan.
3. Have children peel the bananas and then mash them with forks, spoons, or even their hands. They can each mash a banana in a small bowl, then dump the mashed banana into a large mixing bowl.
4. Add the melted butter to the bananas and mix with a wooden spoon. Then mix in the sugar, egg, and vanilla. Preschoolers can do this step.
5. Sprinkle the baking soda and salt over the mixture, then mix them in. Stir in the flour. School-age children can do this step.
6. Pour the batter into the loaf pan and bake for 1 hour. Cool on a rack.

Toasted Banana Treat

Kids will love making this banana treat!

Bread slices (one per child)
Ripe bananas (one per child)
Ground cinnamon

1. Preheat your oven to 450°F.
2. Use your fist to pound the bread slices until they're flattened. Children will love doing this step! Place the pounded bread onto a baking sheet.
3. Slice the bananas. School-age children can do this task with a butter knife. Preschoolers can even do it with a spoon.
4. Place the slices on the bread. Preschoolers and school-age children may want to arrange the slices in a design.
5. Sprinkle cinnamon on the banana slices. Toddlers can help with this task.
6. Bake the bread for 10 minutes or until the bread is toasted to a light brown.

Host Tip
Instead of bananas and cinnamon, try strawberries and honey or blueberries and cream cheese.

Fragrant Cinnamon Buns

These delicious cinnamon buns will delight kids' senses!

2 cups biscuit mix   *Margarine*
⅔ cup milk   *¼ cup sugar*
Flour   *1 teaspoon ground cinnamon*

1. Preheat your oven to 425°F. Toddlers can grease the baking sheet. Unwrap one end of a stick of butter and have the toddler rub it all over the bottom and sides of the sheet.
2. In a small bowl, combine the biscuit mix with the milk until it forms a dough.
3. Gently knead the dough on a floured surface. School-age children will enjoy this step.
4. Roll the dough into an 8-by-12-inch rectangle and spread margarine to cover it completely. This is a good task for preschoolers.
5. In another small bowl, mix the sugar with the cinnamon. Toddlers can do this task. Then sprinkle the mixture on the dough to cover it completely.
6. Roll the dough tightly from one short end to the other, then pinch the ends closed. School-age children can do this step.
7. Cut the rolled dough at 1-inch intervals to make circles, then place them on the greased baking sheet.
8. Bake the dough for 15 minutes. This recipe makes 6 buns.

Host Tip

After they have been baked, cinnamon buns can be stored in your refrigerator for 2–3 weeks and in the freezer for up to 3 months.

Homemade Butter

Let kids move, shake, and wiggle as they make this butter.

1 pint heavy whipping cream
Salt (optional)

1. Pour the cream into a clean 32-ounce jar (a mayonnaise jar works great).
2. Wrap the jar in a dishtowel and secure with a rubber band to prevent the jar from breaking if dropped.
3. Shake the jar 20–30 minutes. Children will enjoy taking turns doing this step. (See next page for fun shaking ideas.) At first, the cream will coat the sides of the jar, but then you will see it pull away from the sides and take on a firmer consistency as it forms lumps of butter.
4. Empty the jar into a colander to separate the butter from the buttermilk. Dispose of the buttermilk, unless you plan to use it for our pancake recipe (see page 351).
5. Put the butter in a bowl and cover it with cold water. Empty the bowl into the colander to rinse the butter. This is to remove any extra buttermilk, which will make your butter taste sour.
6. Put the butter back into the bowl and gently stir in the salt, if you like.
7. Scoop the butter with a spoon into an ice-cube tray and refrigerate for 1 hour. You should have about ½ cup butter or enough to fill at least 6 ice-cube squares halfway.
8. Enjoy the homemade butter on toast, waffles, pancakes, or muffins.

Host Tip

Here are some fun ways for children to shake the jar:

- Have them sit in a circle and roll the jar to one another.
- Have them hop, skip, or jump while holding the jar.
- Put the jar in a backpack, put on some lively music, and have kids dance while taking turns wearing the backpack.
- Set a timer for one minute and have one child shake the jar. When the minute is up, set the timer again and let another child shake the jar for one minute.

Homemade Applesauce

This recipe may be perfect for a baby, and older children will definitely love it, too!

5 medium apples
½ cup water
Pinch of cinnamon

1. Wash the apples, then peel them. Toddlers and preschoolers can help do these tasks, respectively.
2. Core the apples, then dice them. School-age children can do the dicing.
3. Combine the diced apples, water, and cinnamon in a large saucepan and bring to a gentle boil. Lower the heat and simmer for 4 minutes.
4. Use a potato masher to crush the diced apples. Simmer for 2 more minutes until the mixture is the consistency of a sauce.
5. Place in a bowl and allow to cool in the refrigerator overnight. This recipe makes 4–6 cups of applesauce.

S'mores Creatures

Children will love making these tasty creatures! This recipe makes one creature, so adjust the ingredients based on the number of kids (and their hunger!).

2 graham crackers
2 chocolate squares
2 chocolate chips
1 large marshmallow

1. Set a graham cracker on a paper plate, then top with the chocolate squares.
2. Place a marshmallow on top of the chocolate squares. Set the chocolate chips on top of the marshmallow to make eyes.
3. Microwave the creature for 10–15 seconds or until the marshmallow starts to puff up.
4. Remove it from the microwave and watch the creature shrink. Top with another graham cracker and enjoy!

Chapter 11

Seasons & Holidays

During holidays, friends love to gather to eat sugary treats and swap gifts. But I found what they treasure most are the traditions they celebrate.

—Lisa

Celebrating holidays and seasonal changes is a great way to strengthen friendship bonds. In this chapter, we include fun activities that commemorate both traditional and unusual occasions—from Thanksgiving to National Bubble Week. With these themed arts-and-crafts projects, games, and activities, we encourage you to treat each holiday and season as an opportunity to share traditions or create new ones with friends.

Doing the Bubble Pop

Celebrated around the first day of spring, National Bubble Week is the perfect time to play with bubbles.

What You'll Need	All Ages	Babies	Toddlers	Preschoolers	School-Age Children
Nontoxic bubble solution	🖐				
Plastic wands	🖐				
Straws				🖐	🖐
Household objects, such as paper clips, spatulas, paper plates, and so on					🖐
Kiddie pool and Hula-Hoop					🖐

All kids love to blow bubbles! As the playmates have fun blowing bubbles, here's a fun action story to recite together:

I blew a great big bubble. (Blow bubbles.)
It landed on the wand. (Try to catch a bubble on the wand.)
I gave it to my [friend]. (Hand the wand to someone.)
Now it is all gone! (Pop the bubble!)

Babies

Babies will love to track the bubbles as they drift by and eventually pop. When babies are around six months old, they may try to grab the bubbles. To help them "catch" bubbles, wet their hands with the bubble solution, taking care that they don't put it in their mouths. Blow bubbles their way and help the babies hold their hands out to catch them. They may be able to touch the bubbles for a moment before they pop!

Toddlers

Toddlers may be ready to blow their first bubbles. Have them dip the wands into the bubble solution, then slowly pull them out. Show them how to make an O shape with their lips, and then gently blow on the bubble solution. Offer to hold their wand on their first couple of tries.

Preschoolers

Teach preschoolers how to blow a double bubble: Blow a bubble and gently catch it on the wand. Have preschoolers dip a straw into the bubble solution and slowly insert it into the bubble. Because the straw is wet, it shouldn't pop the bubble. Once inside, have them gently blow into the straw. Did they create a double bubble? This experiment may take several tries and will exercise their motor skills, concentration, and patience!

School-Age Children

School-age children can make their own wands from household objects. For instance, they can twist and mold a paper clip to resemble a wand. Other possibilities include straws, spatulas with holes, and plastic plates with holes cut in the bottom. To make the ultimate bubble, take this activity outside. Cover the bottom of a kiddie pool with bubble solution and have them use a Hula-Hoop as a wand!

Host Tip

Run out of bubble solution? Here's how to make a homemade batch: Mix one cup nontoxic dishwashing liquid, two cups water, and two teaspoons sugar.

Did You Know?

National Bubble Week was first celebrated in 2000 and was initiated by OddzOn, makers of Koosh Bubbles. The press release read, "The grassroots 'bubblebration,' to be inaugurated through events in markets around the country, was created to herald the first day of spring—the unspoken first day of the bubble-blowing season."

Signs of Spring

Plastic eggs and natural objects make for a fun guessing game!

What You'll Need	All Ages	Babies	Toddlers	Preschoolers	School-Age Children
Small baskets (or bags)	✋				
Brightly colored plastic eggs	✋				
Cereal		✋			

Give each child a basket and several plastic eggs. Tell them to search outside for small natural objects to put in the eggs, such as small rocks, leaves, grass, pine needles, acorns, bark, puddle water, mud, and more. When the children are done, have them gather for a guessing game. Each child will shake an egg, and the playmates will try to guess its contents. If the object doesn't make a noise when shaken, the child can give the playmates a hint. For example, they can say, "Inside is something squirrels like to eat!" After the playmates have guessed, the child can open the egg carefully to reveal the object.

Babies

The shape and bright colors of plastic eggs will appeal to babies. If the babies are eating solids, fill an egg with cereal. While older playmates hunt for objects to put in their eggs, babies will enjoy shaking their eggs, then eating the snack inside. If babies are not eating solids, give them a tour of the outdoors as you search for objects to put in eggs for them. Point out blossoming flowers, chirping birds, and the blue sky.

Toddlers

Rather than hunt for objects, toddlers may prefer to load and unload their eggs into and out of the baskets. Show them how to pull an egg apart and snap it back together. Encourage them to scoop up small pebbles into eggs. They'll enjoy shaking it during the guessing game.

Preschoolers

Preschoolers will enjoy searching for objects for the guessing game. To challenge them, describe a fairly visible nature object, such as a white rock, and ask them to find it and put it in their eggs.

School-Age Children

School-age children will be busy collecting objects. For a special assignment, give them the task of collecting objects whose names begin with a letter in the word *spring*. For example:

> *Sand*
> *Pine cone*
> *Rock*
> *Insect*
> *Nut (acorn)*
> *Grass*

Host Tip

If the children collect any live insects, ask them not to shake the bugs in their eggs. Instead, gently explore the creatures together before releasing them.

The Great Easter Egg Search

Add your own twist to an outdoor Easter egg hunt!

What You'll Need	All Ages	Babies	Toddlers	Preschoolers	School-Age Children
Plastic eggs (one color per child)	🖐				
Treats for eggs, including love notes, animal crackers, Goldfish crackers, stickers, and so on			🖐	🖐	🖐
Baskets		🖐			
Ribbon		🖐			
Chalk				🖐	🖐

Fill plastic eggs with age-appropriate treats for toddlers, preschoolers, and school-age children. Then hide the eggs around your yard. Designate a different color for each child so children will know which eggs have been filled just for them!

Babies

Babies love to handle colorful plastic eggs. If the babies are older than six months, set them next to small baskets filled with empty eggs. They may take out one egg at a time, or they may decide to dump the basket and fill it up again. If the babies are younger than six months, entertain them with an egg bobber during the

365

egg hunt: Tape a length of ribbon to an empty egg and dangle the egg near the baby's hands, letting her try to grab it.

Toddlers

Place toddlers' eggs in fairly visible locations, then give them baskets, and send them off on the hunt! After they've collected the eggs, help them count the eggs. Encourage toddlers to open and shut the eggs to help build their motor skills—and to find the treats inside.

Preschoolers and School-Age Children

Hide preschoolers' and school-age children's eggs in both easy and challenging locations. Give them baskets, then draw chalk maps to their eggs on the sidewalk or driveway. Provide orientation. For example, say, "This is our house. This is the front porch and the driveway. The eggs I want you to find are right here." Draw an *X* on the location. This activity will help children's ability to follow directions, identify locations, and learn navigation skills. For fun, let the children hide an egg and draw a map for you to find it.

My toddler created his own game with the eggs. He enjoyed opening the eggs and finding the treasures, but he had a hard time closing an egg once it was opened. He decided to put a few treasures on a Frisbee and place the egg halves on top of them. He loved lifting the eggs to find his treasures all over again! For fun, I asked, "Where is the animal cracker?" He lifted each shell until he found the animal cracker.

—Lisa

Cinco de Mayo Piñatas

Celebrate this festive Mexican holiday with homemade piñatas.

What You'll Need	All Ages	Babies	Toddlers	Preschoolers	School-Age Children
Paper lunch bags			✋	✋	✋
Crayons			✋	✋	✋
Fun items, such as soft or plastic toys, age-appropriate candy, and so on			✋	✋	✋
Tape			✋	✋	✋
Rope (or string)			✋	✋	✋
Scarf or handkerchief to use as a blindfold			✋	✋	✋
Plastic bat			✋	✋	✋
Large paper bag		✋			
Baby toy		✋			

Give toddlers, preschoolers, and school-age children each a paper lunch bag to decorate with crayons. When the bags are decorated, help the kids fill them with fun, unbreakable items from around the house, then tape them closed. Hang each piñata by taping a length of rope to it and tying the rope to a clothesline or a low tree branch. One by one, blindfold the children, spin them slowly, then encourage them to try and break open their piñatas with a plastic bat.

Babies

While older playmates make the piñatas, use a large paper bag to entertain babies. For babies six months or older, lay the bag on its side and place favorite toys inside it. Set the babies next to the open end of the bag and encourage them to retrieve the toys. If babies are younger than six months, place them on their tummies and have them use their neck muscles to get a peek inside the bags. For a fun peekaboo game, hide an object under the bag, then lift up the bag quickly to reveal the toy.

Toddlers

At this age, toddlers will enjoy seeing what items fit into the bag just as much as they'll enjoy decorating it. They will probably fill and empty their bags several times. When it's time to break open the piñatas, they may need your assistance with the plastic bat.

Preschoolers and School-Age Children

Encourage preschoolers and school-age children to decorate their piñatas as people, animals, or their favorite characters. They may spend a long time decorating their piñatas and a short time breaking them open!

> **Did You Know?**
> Cinco de Mayo commemorates the victory of Mexican forces on May 5, 1862. Today, Mexicans celebrate the day with parades and speeches.

A Child's Touch Bracelet

This Mother's Day charm bracelet will forever capture each child's unique fingerprint.

What You'll Need	All Ages	Babies	Toddlers	Preschoolers	School-Age Children
Quick-drying molding clay in different colors	✋				
Toothpick	✋				
String	✋				

Let each child choose a color of clay, then flatten a nickel-size piece of each color until it's half an inch thick. Gently press each child's fingerprint into a clay piece, rolling the finger back and forth firmly to capture the print. Use a toothpick to poke a hole in the top of each clay piece, then use the toothpick to inscribe each child's initials on the back of their respective charms. After the clay hardens overnight, help older children thread the pieces onto string to make a bracelet.

Babies

At the beginning of the activity, show the different colors of clay to the babies. Be sure to name each color. Perhaps they will coo or squeal to signal their preferences! Let older playmates decide which colors the babies like best. Before pressing babies' finger-tips into the clay, let them feel it. They will love to explore the texture with their hands, but make sure they don't put the clay into their mouths.

Toddlers, Preschoolers, and School-Age Children

After taking children's fingerprints, ask them to help you choose a safe place for the charms to dry overnight. Then let them play with the remaining clay. Toddlers may just enjoy squeezing and pounding the material, but preschoolers and school-age children may create figures and shapes for Mother's Day presents. Once the clay has hardened overnight, preschoolers and school-age children can help thread the charms onto the string, then help wrap the gift for Mom or another special adult.

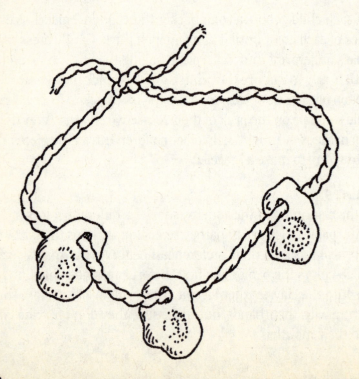

Mother's Day Window Boxes

Children can create a special window box of flowers that will last forever. No need to water!

What You'll Need	All Ages	Babies	Toddlers	Preschoolers	School-Age Children
Scissors	✋				
Cardboard egg cartons	✋				
Play dough	✋				
Pencil		✋	✋	✋	
Construction paper		✋	✋	✋	
Pad of washable ink		✋			
Glue sticks	✋				
Popsicle sticks		✋	✋	✋	
Child-safe scissors				✋	✋
Tissue paper					✋
Pipe cleaners					✋

Cut the lids off the egg cartons, then cut the bottom of each carton in half lengthwise so you have two long rows of egg cups. Each window box requires only one of these rows, so you'll get two window boxes from one egg carton. Put some play dough in each egg cup. Children can then make flowers to "plant" in the play dough.

Babies

To create their flowers, trace around their hands on construction paper and cut the tracings out. To decorate the petals, press their fingertips onto an ink pad, then onto each finger of the cutout. Glue the bloom onto a Popsicle stick. Before you plant the flowers in the carton, hold it up to each baby and count each "petal" out loud. Then take each baby's hand and count each of his fingers to help him make the connection between the flower and his hand.

Toddlers

Cut a circle from construction paper, then cut two triangles into the top to create a tulip. They can then glue Popsicle sticks to the blooms with your help. Toddlers will also enjoy helping you put play dough into the egg cups. Show them how to roll the dough into small balls. Dab glue onto the bottom of each egg cup, then have toddlers place a ball into each.

Preschoolers

For preschoolers' own unique flowers, have them draw different-size circles on a piece of construction paper and cut them out. Using the largest circle as a base, they can glue the other circles slightly overlapping one another to create layered petals. When the bloom is finished, have the preschoolers glue each one onto a Popsicle stick.

School-Age Children

If school-age children want more elaborate flowers, help them follow these steps to make a three-dimensional bloom out of tissue paper:

1. Cut twelve squares, each five inches long and wide, from different-colored tissue paper.
2. Stack the squares in the following pattern: square, diamond, square, diamond, and so on.
3. Place one hand under all the layers of the stack, then lift your index finger to create a peak in the middle.
4. Grasp the peak with the fingers and thumb of your other hand (making sure to grasp all the layers at once), and twist the peak to form a knob.
5. Wrap one end of a pipe cleaner around the knob to create a stem.
6. Lastly, unfurl the tissue paper layers to create petals. Voilà! A beautiful, full flower!

Host Tip

Spray the flowers with a pleasing scent. We recommend lavender to bring a sense of peace and harmony. You can also use perfume.

Patriotic Wreath

Celebrate Memorial Day with this homemade star wreath.

What You'll Need	All Ages	Babies	Toddlers	Preschoolers	School-Age Children
Scissors			🖐	🖐	🖐
White construction paper			🖐	🖐	🖐
Cotton balls	🖐				
Red tissue paper	🖐				
Blue painter's tape	🖐				
Glue stick			🖐	🖐	🖐
Paper plate			🖐	🖐	🖐

Prepare for this activity by cutting out nine stars, four inches across, from white construction paper. Give toddlers, preschoolers, and school-age children three stars each and instruct each of them to decorate one star with white cotton balls, one with red tissue paper, and one with blue painter's tape. When they are done, help them glue the finished stars around the edge of a paper plate to create a patriotic wreath.

Babies

Let babies explore the art supplies on their highchair trays while their playmates decorate their stars. Babies will enjoy the soft cotton balls, the crinkly tissue paper, and the sticky painter's tape. When the wreath is finished, have the older children show it to the babies—they will enjoy gazing at the colors and patterns.

Toddlers

Assist toddlers with their stars. For the white and red stars, dab glue on the cotton balls and pieces of tissue paper, then let the toddlers press them onto the stars. For the blue stars, tear off small pieces of tape and let toddlers pull the pieces from your fingers and press them onto the stars.

Preschoolers

After everyone has decorated their stars, preschoolers may enjoy picking a pattern for gluing them onto the paper plate. For example, one may suggest that the blue stars go together, followed by the red ones, and then the white ones. Or one may suggest alternating individual red, white, and blue stars around the plate.

School-Age Children

Show school-age children how to make a textured star. They can roll the tissue paper into small balls, dot them with glue, and place them close together on the star. They can also pull apart the cotton balls slightly, then press them onto a glue-covered star to create a wispy look. Lastly, they can create squares across the stars with the tape.

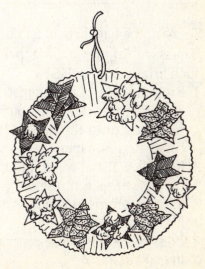

Wave That Flag

Proudly creating a homemade American flag as a group is a great way to celebrate Flag Day.

What You'll Need	All Ages	Babies	Toddlers	Preschoolers	School-Age Children
Large blue and white sheets of construction paper	✋				
Child-safe scissors	✋				
Glue stick	✋				
Red and yellow tissue paper	✋				
Paintbrush	✋				
Watered-down glue (2 parts water to 1 part glue)	✋				
Marker	✋				

To make the flag, help older children follow these instructions. Babies will enjoy watching their playmates busily work with such bright art supplies!

1. From a sheet of blue construction paper, cut a rectangle roughly a quarter of the size of the sheet. Glue the rectangle onto the upper-left corner of a white sheet of construction paper.
2. Rip yellow tissue paper into twenty small pieces and tear red tissue paper into seven long strips.
3. Use a paintbrush to apply watered-down glue all over the flag.
4. Press the yellow tissue paper pieces onto the blue rectangle to make stars.

5. Starting at the bottom of the sheet, lay the red tissue paper strips horizontally at equal distances on the white part of the flag. Trim the top strips to accommodate the blue rectangle.
6. To preserve the flag (and add shine), brush watered-down glue on the tissue paper.
7. After the glue has dried, use a marker to record words that the children use to describe their country and the people who protect it.

As you make the flag together, consider doing the following activities:

- Sing patriotic songs like "The Star-Spangled Banner" and "You're a Grand Old Flag." Younger children will love hearing everyone's voices and may try to "sing" along!

- Explain the significance of the stars and stripes on the American flag. Point out that while your homemade flag has twenty stars, the real flag has fifty—one for each state.

- Provide a world map or globe and point out the United States. Then point out your state and town. Encourage the children to explore the other countries on the map. Introducing geography to children at an early age will heighten their curiosity about the great big world!

- Look through books or magazines with colorful pictures of the United States. Identify the landmarks and encourage children to point to objects or shapes they recognize. (While looking at pictures of American locations, note those you want to visit with your families. Enjoy your freedom to do so!)

Day in the Life of Daddy

On Father's Day, playmates can pay tribute to their dads or father figures with special performances!

What You'll Need	All Ages	Babies	Toddlers	Preschoolers	School-Age Children
A few of Dad's shirts, ties, hats, and shoes	✋				

Before the playdate, tell the playgroup they're going to perform a show about their dads or special father figures. Ask each of them what they love to do with Dad, and have them recall the tasks Dad does every day (for example, shaving his face or mowing the lawn). Have them each choose (or help them choose) one of those tasks or actions to perform, as well as bring any props along such as Dad's ties or shirts. When the audience and performers are ready, let the show begin! Remember to tape it so all dads can watch later!

Babies

Babies can look the part by wearing one of Dad's hats. For babies who are old enough to play an interactive game with Dad, like rolling a ball back and forth, have one of the older children play the baby's part, and let "Dad" and "the baby" roll the ball to each other.

Toddlers

Toddlers will love dressing up in Dad's shirt and tie. When it's their turn to perform, have them do something they associate doing with their dad. For example, for toddlers who like to cut a rug together with their dad, turn on Dad's favorite music and let them dance. Or, for toddlers who enjoy story time with their dad, have them "read" a favorite book to their teddy bear.

Preschoolers

Preschoolers may enjoy walking in their dads' shoes. Let them reenact parts of Dad's day according to his different shoes. For example, while wearing Dad's dressy work shoes, a preschooler can pretend to type on a computer and answer the phone. Then the preschooler can put on Dad's sneakers and pretend to mow the lawn.

School-Age Children

School-age children can reenact an entire sequence of events in their dad's daily life. For example, they can put on pair of Dad's pajamas, then pretend to shave, change into work clothes, comb their hair, read the paper, drink a cup of coffee, let out the dog, kiss the kids goodbye, and more.

Summer Solstice Sun Catchers

Make colorful sun catchers to greet the summer sunshine on the longest day of the year!

What You'll Need	All Ages	Babies	Toddlers	Preschoolers	School-Age Children
Clear contact paper		✋	✋		
Colored tissue paper		✋	✋		✋
Scissors		✋	✋		
Clear plastic lids from deli containers, to-go tubs, and so on				✋	✋
Permanent markers in at least three colors				✋	✋
Yarn or ribbon					✋
Child-safe scissors					✋
Hole punch					✋

While you create sun catchers for babies and toddlers, older kids can make their own. Hang the finished sun catchers with yarn near a light source and watch the colors dance!

Babies

If a baby is six months or older, give him a sheet of clear contact paper to touch. He'll enjoy the sticky sensation. Afterward, lay ripped-up pieces of light-colored tissue paper on the contact paper and cover them with another sheet of contact paper.

Cut out a shape for his very own sun catcher. The dazzling colors will delight a baby, no matter what his age!

Toddlers

Set a sheet of contact paper sticky side up in front of toddlers and have them press a piece of tissue paper onto it. Stick a second piece of tissue paper so it overlaps the first piece, and show toddlers how to hold the contact paper up to the light to see the colors glow. Encourage them to overlap different colors of paper in pairs to create new colors—red over blue makes purple, and yellow over red makes orange. When finished, place another sheet of contact paper on the tissue paper, then ask them what shape they'd like you to cut out for the final sun catcher. Toddlers can then help you find the perfect spot to hang it.

Preschoolers

Give each preschooler a large, clear plastic lid and encourage them to color one side of it completely. Show them how to make colored spirals by drawing one continuous spiral that begins around the perimeter of the lid and then becomes smaller and smaller as it reaches the center. If they like, they can switch the color of marker along the way.

School-Age Children

Begin with the directions for preschoolers but have them further decorate their sun catcher by adding colorful tails to the bottom. Have them cut ribbons, yarn, or thin strips of tissue paper in various lengths. Secure them to each catcher, using a hole punch to create holes at the base of the lid, and tie the decorations to it.

Seashell Magnets

Nothing says summer like seashells, so use them to create magnets kids can enjoy season after season.

What You'll Need	All Ages	Babies	Toddlers	Preschoolers	School-Age Children
Seashells (from beach or local craft store)	✋				
Sponges or old toothbrushes			✋	✋	✋
Washable tempera paint and paintbrush			✋	✋	✋
Mineral or baby oil			✋	✋	✋
Magnetic tape			✋	✋	✋
Quick-drying glue		✋			
Empty egg carton		✋			
School glue				✋	✋
Construction paper				✋	✋
Child-safe scissors				✋	✋

To begin, show any older children how to gently clean the seashells with water and a sponge or old toothbrush. When the shells are dry, children can decorate them with paint. If the kids prefer a natural look, they can use their fingers to wipe the shells with mineral or baby oil to make them shine. When they are done, affix magnetic tape to the back of each shell.

Babies

Seashells have many different textures, which make them attractive to curious babies' hands. For safe exploration, glue clean seashells without jagged edges into the cups of an empty egg carton. For an auditory experience, hold a large seashell to babies' ears. Do they react to the sound?

Toddlers

Toddlers will enjoy exploring large seashells (smaller ones pose a choking hazard) before they paint them. Can they hear noises when they hold shells to their ears? Have them describe what each shell feels like. Is it bumpy or smooth? What color is it?

Preschoolers and School-Age Children

Preschoolers and school-age children can create seashell animals. To make a dog, for example, they can paint on eyes and a mouth. They can then glue a small pair of brown construction-paper triangles to the top of the shell for ears and a small brown strip on the bottom for a tail.

Host Tip
To learn more about shells, read with the kids the delightful picture book *Shells! Shells! Shells!* by Nancy Elizabeth Wallace.

Grandparents Day Video

Create a special video displaying each child's accomplishments for their grandparents or "grandfriends."

What You'll Need	All Ages	Babies	Toddlers	Preschoolers	School-Age Children
Camcorder	✋				
Children displaying their talents!	✋				

Grab the camcorder and tell the children you will record a special video for their grandparents. Let the children decide what they would like to do on the video. Some age-appropriate suggestions are below.

Babies
Be sure to get a close-up of each baby, noting any characteristics that bear a resemblance to those of the baby's grandparents. Try to capture smiles by singing favorite song or having a playmate play peekaboo with the baby. Any older children can serve as "directors," encouraging the baby to show off such recent accomplishments as sitting up or rolling over.

Toddlers
Toddlers are beginning to gain more control of their art projects. Record their coloring or creating other artwork that you can send along with the video. Ask toddlers to describe the artwork on camera for their grandparents.

Preschoolers

Preschoolers are learning about the letters in their names, and they may even be able to write them for their proud grandparents. You can also record any thoughts or special memories of times they have enjoyed with their grandparents.

School-Age Children

Interview school-age children about their favorite sports, classes at school, and friendships. Try to ask open-ended questions. They may also want to write and recite a poem about how special their grandparents are to them.

Did You Know?
In 1978, President Jimmy Carter proclaimed that National Grandparents Day would be celebrated every year on the first Sunday after Labor Day.

Apple Taste Test

Autumn is the perfect time to taste all kinds of apples!

What You'll Need	All Ages	Babies	Toddlers	Preschoolers	School-Age Children
Several different kinds of apples, such as Granny Smith, McIntosh, and Golden Delicious	🖐				
Paring knife and fork					
Paper					🖐
Pencil					🖐

If possible, take kids to a local apple orchard and pick a variety of apples together. If visiting an orchard isn't possible, buy various kinds of apples at the supermarket. At home, gather the children for a taste test. Before eating the apples, any older kids can examine them and describe their differences. Then serve a piece of each apple to each child (in age-appropriate servings). Discuss its taste and have school-age children record younger children's votes on a special chart.

Babies

If babies are eating fruit, their vote counts, too! Have them try a tiny bit of each apple after it's been peeled, sliced, and mashed with a fork. (Start with McIntosh because of its sweet taste.) Do they enjoy it? Have the other children decide. If babies aren't eating fruits, have a playmate hold an apple slice in front of them to see if they react to its color and smell. Record a coo or smile on the chart!

Toddlers

Give each toddler a few bite-size pieces of the different apples. Even the pickiest toddler will likely try apples, although some toddlers may show you they don't care for a specific variety by spitting it out! This activity is also a great opportunity to teach colors. Help toddlers identify the color of each apple.

Preschoolers

Have preschoolers try each apple variety sliced or whole, with or without the peel. Adjectives are becoming a huge part of their vocabulary. Use this activity to encourage them to describe the look and taste of each apple. For example, they may use words like *sweet, crunchy, soft*, or *chewy* to express their thoughts.

School-Age Children

School-age children can create a taste-test chart like the one shown below. They can list the name of each apple variety down a sheet of paper, then record each taster's name across the top. As each child tastes each apple, school-age children can record responses with a smiley face or a frowning face. Don't let them forget to taste the apples themselves and record their own reactions!

Sample Taste-Test Chart				
	Jake	Brooke	Kyle	Noah
McIntosh	☺	☹	☺	☹
Granny Smith	☹	☺	☹	☺
Golden Delicious	☺	☹	☺	☺

Leaf Place Mats

Autumn leaves will make beautiful place settings!

What You'll Need	All Ages	Babies	Toddlers	Preschoolers	School-Age Children
Fallen leaves	✋				
Scissors	✋				
Paper grocery bags	✋				
Glue sticks		✋	✋		
Washable tempera paint				✋	✋
Paintbrushes				✋	✋
Clear contact paper	✋				
Ribbon and hole punch		✋			
Crayons					✋

On a pleasant autumn day, playmates can gather a variety of fallen leaves. When inside, cut paper grocery bags into eight-inch-by-eleven-inch rectangles for toddlers, preschoolers, and school-age children. Children can then glue leaves onto these homemade place mats or lightly paint a leaf and press the imprint onto their paper rectangles. When the finished place mats are dry, cover them with clear contact paper and trim the excess.

Babies

As older children make the place mats, make each baby a bib from the same materials. Cut a bib shape from a paper bag. Show the babies some brightly colored leaves and describe their colors: "This leaf is yellow; this leaf is orange." See if they coo or reach for their favorites. Glue the leaves to the bibs, cover each bib with contact paper, and use ribbon and a hole punch to secure the bib around a baby's neck. (Babies should wear the bib only under your close supervision.)

Toddlers

Toddlers may enjoy gluing leaves onto the grocery bag with your help, but they may have an easier time creating their place mats if you skip the bag altogether. Instead, tape an eight-inch-by-eleven-inch sheet of clear contact paper sticky side up to the table and encourage them to stick the leaves directly to it. During this process, however, toddlers may discover that the dried leaves will often crumble if they try to pull them off the contact paper or if they press them on too roughly. If this happens, talk about cause and effect—and make sure they have lots of leaves! When they're done, cover their work with another sheet of contact paper.

Preschoolers

At this age, preschoolers have the dexterity to paint one side of a leaf and press it onto their place mat. Encourage them to use different colors of paint and different shapes of leaves to create a design.

School-Age Children

For an added art challenge, encourage school-age children to incorporate the leaf imprints into a drawing on their place mats. For instance, they can turn an imprint of a maple leaf into butterfly wings or an imprint of an oak leaf into the flames from a rocket.

Columbus Day Sailing Hats

To commemorate Christopher Columbus's voyage to America, set sail for fun with these easy-to-make sailor hats!

What You'll Need	All Ages	Babies	Toddlers	Preschoolers	School-Age Children
Newspaper	🖐				
Tape	🖐				
Decorations, including crayons, stickers, glue, feathers, and strips of colored paper	🖐				
Toy boat			🖐		
Empty paper towel roll				🖐	

From an old newspaper, pull out a spread (four pages, front and back) for each child. Older children can help you fold the paper into sailing hats for themselves and their younger play-mates. Here's how:

1. Close the spread at the vertical crease and turn the paper sideways so the open edge is on the bottom and the crease is at the top.
2. Fold down the top corners so they meet, then tape them together.
3. Fold the bottom edge up several inches all around the paper. (This may take several tries.)

4. Decorate the hat with crayons, stickers, feathers, and colored paper strips.

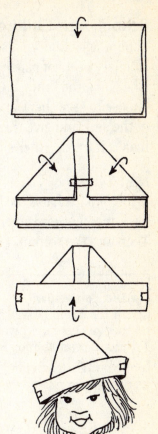

Babies

When the babies' hats are done, place them on their heads, then seat the babies face-out on laps and sing the song "Row, Row, Row Your Boat" with them. If you like, sing this fun version to the tune:

> *Sail, sail, sail your boat*
> *in the ocean blue.*
> *Merrily, merrily, Columbus sailed*
> *in 1492.*

Toddlers

While wearing their hats, toddlers can pretend to be real sailors. Fill the kitchen sink or the bathtub and let them float toy boats in it. Ask them about their sailing adventures: "Where is your boat going? Is your boat going slow or fast?"

Preschoolers

To be a true explorer of the time, preschoolers should have their own telescopes. Let them decorate empty paper towel rolls with stickers. Encourage them to use their imaginations to locate objects at sea with their telescopes.

School-Age Children

School-age children also can make three smaller hats from smaller sheets of paper to represent Columbus's three ships (the Niña, the Pinta, and the Santa Maria). Perhaps they'll choose to race them in the sink! Line up the ships on one side of the sink and give them each a gentle shove. Which one makes it to the other side first?

Host Tip

If you find the hat is too big and falling over a child's face, simply place it on his head and pinch the back to create the ideal size. Then tape the bottom of the hat where you pinched it.

> **Did You Know?**
> In his famed 1492 voyage, Columbus didn't set out to prove the world was round—people already knew Earth was round. Rather, he was attempting to find a route to the Far East.

Spider Games

Build a big, soft spider for some active Halloween games!

What You'll Need	All Ages	Babies	Toddlers	Preschoolers	School-Age Children
Several large pillows	🖐				
8 large towels	🖐				

To create the spider's body, help the children pile pillows in the center of a room with lots of open space. Then roll up the towels and place them around the pillow pile to create the spider's eight legs. Have each child sit on a spider leg (hold a baby in your lap as you sit on a leg) to play these games.

The Laughing Spider
Recite the following story together while tickling the spider legs:

*This great big spider
has ticklish legs.
So we tickled,
and he laughed.
And then this great big spider
told us to jump into the bath!*
(Everyone jumps onto the spider's body!)

Creepy, Creepy Spider
Have everyone sit in a circle. Choose one child to walk around the circle and tap each playmate she passes on the shoulder. As she does so, everyone recites:

Creepy, creepy spider,
climbing in the webs,
tapped me on the shoulder—
I guess it's time for bed!

At the word *bed*, the last person tapped is out of the game and must move to the spider's body. Play again until there are no more shoulders to tap. Then choose a new person to tap shoulders.

Babies

When it's time to jump onto the spider's body during each game, gently move onto the pillows with each baby. The motion will excite them! The spider also creates a great tummy-time experience for babies: Lay their chests over rolled-up towels while supporting their hips. (If babies do tummy time during "Creepy, Creepy Spider," you may want to move their towels far enough away so babies are safe from the action but still close enough to watch playmates play.)

Toddlers

Before playing the games, let toddlers explore the spider legs. Encourage them to first step over the legs while you count them. On their next trip around, have them hold your hands while jumping over the legs and counting them with you. Come up with other ways to travel over the legs. These exercises will strengthen their coordination and muscles.

Preschoolers

Let preschoolers take a leadership role during these games by encouraging them to keep the spider ready for action. They can make sure the legs are in place and the pillows are fluffed. They can also make sure everyone has a turn to tap shoulders during "Creepy, Creepy Spider."

School-Age Children

Instead of tickling the spider legs during "The Laughing Spider" game, school-age children can show off their agility skills by jumping back and forth over their spider leg. Can they do this for the whole song?

After making a spider, the playmates decided to make other creatures with the materials, like a turtle and butterfly.

—Lisa

Pumpkin Faces

Who needs jack-o'-lanterns when you can make paper pump-kin faces?

What You'll Need	All Ages	Babies	Toddlers	Preschoolers	School-Age Children
Child-safe scissors	🖐				
Orange and black construction paper	🖐				
Glue stick	🖐				
Clear contact paper	🖐				

Help the children cut large ovals from orange construction paper—one oval for each baby and three each per toddler, pre-schooler, and school-age child. Also cut out triangles, circles, and squares from black construction paper—one set of shapes for each baby plus at least ten of each shape for each older child. Children then can use the shapes as eyes, noses, mouths, and ears to turn the ovals into pumpkin faces, and you can create a face for the babies to explore.

Babies

Make a pumpkin face for each baby by gluing the shapes onto the oval, then cover it with clear contact paper. The contrast between orange and black will heighten babies' developing sense of color. Let them handle the pumpkin face while you point out its eyes, nose, and mouth, or ask them to point the parts out if they're old enough to identify facial features.

Toddlers
Use this activity to review shapes with toddlers. Work alongside them as they decide which shapes to use for their pumpkin faces. They may want triangles or circles for eyes, for example. Dab glue on the pumpkin and let them press their shapes onto the glue.

Preschoolers
Preschoolers understand the proper placement of facial features, but use this activity to encourage them to work abstractly. For example, they may use a circle for one eye and a square for the other. When their faces are complete, discuss the differences or similarities among them.

School-Age Children
Before school-age children decorate their pumpkin faces, challenge them to turn the art projects into a math project: Given the number of different shapes, how many combinations for eyes can they make (two circles, one circle and one square, two squares, and so on)? Encourage them to work out the problem by creating each combination of shapes on their pumpkins.

Spooky Chairs

These scary chair covers will create the perfect Halloween ambience for a kitchen or a dining room.

What You'll Need	All Ages	Babies	Toddlers	Preschoolers	School-Age Children
Old pillowcases	🖐				
White, black, or orange acrylic paint		🖐			🖐
Paintbrush		🖐			🖐
Wet wipes		🖐			
Fabric markers		🖐		🖐	🖐
Safety pins or masking tape		🖐			
Halloween foam stickers (available at craft stores)			🖐		🖐
Cotton balls			🖐		🖐
Tacky glue			🖐	🖐	🖐
Chalk				🖐	🖐
Black felt				🖐	🖐
Scissors				🖐	🖐

Your playgroup will have a ghoulishly good time decorating one side of their pillowcases. When they're done, slip each pillowcase over the back of a chair so the decorated side is facing out behind the chair.

Babies

Babies can help design pillowcases to decorate the back of their highchairs. Cover the palm side of one of their hands with white paint, then gently press it onto a dark-colored pillowcase several times to make skeletal handprints. If you have only a light-colored pillowcase, paint the babies' palms (not their fingers) orange and press them onto the pillowcases to make pumpkins. Clean their hands with wet wipes when you're done. After the paint has dried, turn the pumpkins into jack-o'-lanterns by drawing features with a fabric marker. When it's complete, affix each pillowcase to the back of a high-chair with safety pins (if the seat is cloth covered) or masking tape (if the seat is plastic).

Toddlers

Toddlers will enjoy decorating their pillowcases with Halloween-themed foam stickers, which may be easier for them to manipulate than regular stickers. They may need help peeling the backs off the stickers, but let them decide where to place the stickers. With your help, they can also create ghosts using cotton balls and tacky glue. Simply pull the cotton balls apart so they are wispy.

Preschoolers

Preschoolers can use chalk to draw spooky shapes on black felt, like a haunted house, witch hat, or bat. Cut out the shapes for them, and let them glue the shapes onto their pillowcases. Have them write their names on their creations with fabric markers.

School-Age Children

With felt, paint, cotton balls, stickers, chalk, and fabric markers, school-age children will have lots of ways to decorate their pillowcases. Encourage them to use the entire pillowcase to create a graveyard scene or haunted house.

Host Tip

If the pillowcases don't fit over your chairs, cut the decorated side from each pillowcase. Cut two strips of fabric just long enough to go around the back of a chair, then safety-pin one strip at the top of the decorated pillowcase piece and the other strip at the bottom to secure it to the chair.

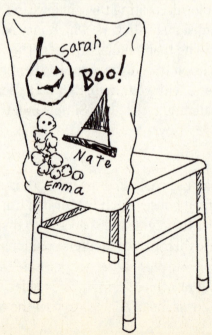

Rock Pumpkins

Create a patch of rock pumpkins for everyone's yard!

What You'll Need	All Ages	Babies	Toddlers	Preschoolers	School-Age Children
Baseball-size rocks	🖐				
Orange paint	🖐				
Zip-close plastic bag		🖐			
Black markers	🖐				
Disposable plastic container			🖐		
Paintbrushes				🖐	🖐
Twigs					🖐
Green paint					🖐
Tacky glue					🖐

Take the playgroup to a park or beach and collect several base-
ball-size rocks. (If necessary, purchase rocks from a craft store
or landscaping center.) At home, rinse the rocks with warm
water and let them dry. Then have the group paint the rocks
orange and use markers to turn them into jack-o'-lanterns.
When finished, each child can bring their rock pumpkins
home to display in their yard.

Babies

Babies can "paint" rocks, too. Pour orange paint into a zip-
close plastic bag and place three rocks inside it. Securely tape
the bag closed. For babies six months or older, help them roll
and shake the rocks inside the bag to coat the rocks with

paint. If they are younger than six months, sit close to them so they can watch you roll and shake the bag. The brightly colored paint will catch babies' attention. Finish by adding jack-o'-lantern features with a marker.

Toddlers

Given their increasing mastery of picking up items, toddlers will enjoy collecting rocks. To help them paint their rocks back home, pour paint into a disposable plastic container. They can carefully drop all of their rocks in the paint and roll them around to paint them on all sides. When the paint is dry, have them tell you what expression you should draw on their pumpkins, or let them draw on the pumpkins themselves.

Preschoolers

As you collect the rocks, encourage preschoolers to find ones that suit their fancy. Do they like bumpy or smooth ones? Tall or short ones? Skinny or fat ones? Their dexterity is becoming more controlled, so when they decorate the jack-o'-lanterns, challenge them to take their time with the paintbrushes and markers.

School-Age Children

School-age children will put a lot of detail into painting their jack-o'-lanterns and drawing the features. As an added touch, they can paint little pieces of twigs green and then glue them as stems onto the tops of their jack-o'-lanterns. They may also want to glue stems onto their playmates' jack-o'-lanterns.

Thanks and Giving

During the Thanksgiving season, serve a helping of love and appreciation with this simple sharing game.

What You'll Need	All Ages	Babies	Toddlers	Preschoolers	School-Age Children
Scarf (or other cloth item)	✋				

You can play this game anytime, but it's especially nice as your group anticipates the Thanksgiving holiday. To play, hand a scarf to one child and ask him to announce something for which he is thankful. Then have him compliment the person sitting to his left and give her the scarf. She then gives thanks and compliments the person on her left while passing on the scarf. The game ends when everyone has given thanks and compliments.

Babies

When it's the baby's turn to receive the scarf, let her hold it while you give thanks and compliment her neighbor on her behalf. For instance, you may say, "The baby is thankful for all the kisses she receives, and she loves playtime!" Tickle her with the scarf to entice a smile for her playmates.

Toddlers

At this age, toddlers' world revolves mostly around their own wants and needs. This game will introduce toddlers to gratitude and appreciation of others. Help them articulate their thankfulness by asking questions such as, "Are you thankful that it was sunny out today so you could play in the yard?" Use similar prompts to help toddlers compliment their neighbors.

Preschoolers

Preschoolers may express thanks for seemingly trivial items like toys or books, but these things bring them joy. Resist leading their responses. Receiving compliments may be preschoolers' favorite part of the game. They are becoming aware of other people's feelings about them and will love hearing that they are important members of the group.

School-Age Children

In this sharing time, ask the school-age children to share something positive and appreciative about all their playmates, rather than just the person on their left. This exercise will hopefully strengthen the friendship bonds.

Host Tip
Don't forget that you get a turn, too. Make sure you compliment each child. They'll love to hear your praise!

Handprint Menorahs

Children can use their handprints to create a menorah—an eight-branch candleholder used to celebrate the Jewish holiday of Hanukkah, the festival of lights.

What You'll Need	All Ages	Babies	Toddlers	Preschoolers	School-Age Children
Construction paper	✋				
Paintbrush	✋				
Washable tempera paint	✋				
Wet wipes	✋				
Crayons				✋	✋
Child-safe scissors				✋	✋
Glue stick				✋	✋

Give each child a sheet of construction paper. Use a paintbrush to lightly paint the palm side of their hands. Have them press one hand onto the paper and then press the other hand next to it so the thumbs overlap. The eight fingers represent candles, which in turn represent the eight nights of Hanukkah. The overlapping thumbprints represent the shamash, the special candle used to light the others. When the children are done, clean their hands with wet wipes.

Babies

After you've made a menorah with the baby's hands, let the baby enjoying making additional handprints on another sheet of paper with the paint remaining on her hands. Babies will likely slap and bang their hands onto the paper to make a delightfully loud noise. See if they'll slap their hands in response after you slap down your hands. Just be sure babies don't put their painted hands in their mouths.

Toddlers
Toddlers are learning about numbers and counting. As you make their menorahs, count the candles together, forward and backward.

Preschoolers and School-Age Children
To prepare for "lighting" the candles on the nights ahead, preschoolers and school-age children can team up to draw and cut out small triangle "flames" from yellow construction paper. They will need nine triangles for each playmate's menorah. When they're done, have them glue a flame to the shamash on each menorah. Then on each night of Hanukkah, they can glue a flame to another candle on their menorahs, starting with the candle on the far right.

Host Tip
Teach children the history of Hanukkah and the menorah. Here are some great books to read together: *It's Hanukkah!* by Santiago Cohen, *Festival of Lights: The Story of Hanukkah* by Maida Silverman, and *Hanukkah, Oh Hanukkah* by Susan L. Roth.

Dreidel Animals

The group will act like animals with this "spin" on a traditional Jewish game!

What You'll Need	All Ages	Babies	Toddlers	Preschoolers	School-Age Children
Paper and pencil	✋				
Dreidel (or see how to make one at the end of this activity)	✋				

Have the group come up with as many animals whose names begin with the letters *G*, *H*, and *S* as they can. Jot down their answers on a sheet of paper. Here are some ideas:

- *G*: Giraffe, grasshopper, gazelle, goat, goose
- *H*: Horse, hummingbird, hawk, hippopotamus
- *S*: Snake, sheep, seal, spider, swan

Next, sit in a circle around a hard surface and take turns spinning a dreidel. Tell the children that when the dreidel stops face-up on *G*, *H*, or *S*, the person who spun it must move and sound like an animal that begins with that letter. For example, if the *G* is face-up, the spinner can honk and move like a goose. Use your list of animals to provide ideas, if necessary. To make the game more challenging, when the *N* is face-up, the spinner may move and sound like any animal he chooses. After the spinner has acted like an animal for at least ten seconds, the others may try to identify the animal, then copy the movements and sounds!

Babies

Spin the dreidel for the babies and help them move like the appropriate animal. For instance, if the *H* lands face-up and you choose a horse, hold the baby face-out against your chest (supporting his head and neck) while you gallop around. Babies will love the action! If you like, make the appropriate animal sounds as well.

Toddlers

Help toddlers spin the dreidel. Or have them hold the dreidel with both hands, shake it, then drop it to reveal a letter. Help toddlers identify the face-up letter, whisper the names of two animals that begin with that letter, then let them choose one to act out.

Preschoolers and School-Age Children

As a challenge, ask preschoolers and school-age children to give the other players hints rather than act like animals during a few of their turns. For instance, a preschooler may say, "This animal likes to eat hay" (horse). A school-age child may say, "The animal I am thinking of can fly backward!" (hummingbird).

Homemade Dreidel

Single-serving milk or juice
  carton
Tape
Plain paper
Pen or marker
Scissors
¼-inch dowel or unsharpened
  pencil

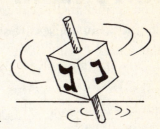

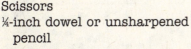

Flatten the top of the carton and tape it down
securely. Cover the carton with plain paper. On each
side, write one of the letters *N, G, H,* and *S* to represent the first letters in the four words of the Hebrew
message *nes gadol hayah sham,* which means "A
great miracle happened there." (Hebrew characters
are read from right to left.)

Poke a small hole in the centers of the top and
bottom of the carton and push the dowel or pencil
through both holes to make a spinning top.

These directions are adapted from *The Arts and
Crafts Busy Book* by Trish Kuffner (Meadowbrook
Press, 2003).

Merry Mini-Houses

These tiny, tasty houses are sure to get kids in the holiday mood!

What You'll Need	All Ages	Babies	Toddlers	Preschoolers	School-Age Children
Wax paper			✋	✋	✋
Paintbrushes and small bowls			✋	✋	✋
Icing (recipe below)			✋	✋	✋
Graham crackers	✋				
Edible decorations, including cereal, fruit snacks, diced fruit, and so on		✋			
Yogurt	✋				

To prepare, make the icing with the recipe provided at the end of this activity. Then lay wax paper in front of any toddlers, preschoolers, and school-age children in your group to use as a workspace. Give them each a paintbrush and a small bowl of icing. Show the group how to use the icing to glue together four graham cracker halves to make the walls of a house. Add two graham cracker halves at a slant to create a roof for the house. Finally, have them decorate the houses by attaching cereal, fruit snacks, diced fruit, and other edible items with the icing. Let the icing harden before displaying (or eating!) the mini-houses.

Babies

As older playmates build their mini-houses, make a mini-creation babies can enjoy: Spread some yogurt on a graham cracker and decorate it with diced fruit. As babies watch their playmates build with the graham crackers, they'll try to do the same. If babies are not eating solids yet, supervise closely if they try to put the items in their mouth. Chances are, they'll be too busy playing to eat!

Toddlers

Although you will likely build the toddlers' mini-houses, they can do the decorating. Show them how to gently paint icing onto the house and stick decorations onto it. A house with a flat roof may make an easier surface for them to decorate.

Preschoolers and School-Age Children

Encourage preschoolers and school-age children to decorate their mini-houses in detail. For example, they can create the outlines of doors or window frames with the small cereal pieces. They can make a walkway, chimney, and more!

Icing Recipe
1 pound confectioner's sugar
¼ teaspoon cream of tartar
3 egg whites

Slowly beat together the sugar, cream of tartar, and egg whites until stiff peaks form.

Rudolph Says

Gather the kids for this game of Simon Says with a Christmas twist.

What You'll Need	All Ages	Babies	Toddlers	Preschoolers	School-Age Children
Red construction paper	🖐				
Scissors	🖐				
Non-petroleum jelly	🖐				

In a room with a lot of open space, tell the group how to play this game: Instead of Simon Says, it's Rudolph the Red-Nosed Reindeer Says. Rudolph will make a command, such as, "Put your hand on your head," "Jump up and down," "Turn around in a circle," and so on. Everyone else must follow the command, but only if Rudolph prefaces it with "Rudolph says…" If Rudolph doesn't say this preface, everyone else must stay still. Affix a small red circle of construction paper to each Rudolph's nose with a dab of non-petroleum jelly. Play the game until each child has had a chance to be Rudolph.

Babies and Toddlers

With your help, babies and toddlers can follow the commands. Toddlers will probably do the action regardless of whether Rudolph prefaces the command with "Rudolph says…" That's okay. At this age, they may not understand the nuances of the game, but it's still good for them to practice following an explicit command!

When it's their turn to be Rudolph, the red circle on the nose will fascinate little ones. Be sure to let them see themselves as Rudolph in a mirror. While you'll have to give commands for a baby Rudolph, toddler Rudolphs will likely love to tell their playmates what to do. Prompt older kids to do the action even if toddlers don't preface their command with "Rudolph says…"

Preschoolers and School-Age Children

This game is a great way for preschoolers and school-age children to practice their listening skills. See how well they can follow the rules. When it's their turn to be Rudolph, encourage them to give commands that reflect Christmas or winter activities. For example, "Pretend to wrap gifts," or, "Sing 'Rudolph the Red-Nosed Reindeer.'"

Did You Know?
The tale of "Rudolph the Red-Nosed Reindeer" was first told in 1939. Ever since, children around the world have looked for his red nose leading Santa's sleigh in the dark sky on Christmas Eve.

A Handful of Christmas

Spread the holiday cheer with this handprint Christmas tree.

What You'll Need	All Ages	Babies	Toddlers	Preschoolers	School-Age Children
Green construction paper	✋				
Pencil	✋				
Child-safe scissors	✋				
Large sheet of white paper	✋				
Star stickers			✋	✋	✋
Glue and tinsel			✋	✋	✋

Help the group trace their hands on green construction paper and cut out the tracings. To complete the tree, you'll need twenty-one hand cutouts, so enlist the help of older children with this step! Show older children how to glue the cutouts (fingers pointing up) onto a large sheet of white paper in six rows of descending number. That is, they will glue a row of six hands along the bottom, then a row of five hands above and slightly overlapping the row of six, then a row of four hands slightly overlapping the row of five, and so on.

Babies

As you trace the baby's hand, recite the following action poem:

> *This little elf's family is as happy as can be, be, be.*
> (Trace the thumb.)
> *They are all full of glee, glee, glee.*
> (Trace the index finger.)

"Yes," the family cheered, "We, we, we
   (Trace the middle finger.)
Have been waiting since you were born, born, born
   (Trace the ring finger.)
To say, 'Wake up! It's Christmas morn, morn, morn!'"
   (Trace the pinky.)

Toddlers, Preschoolers, and School-Age Children

When the tree is complete, they can decorate it with star stickers and also glue on some tinsel. To create special ornaments, have them each cut out a circle from colored construction paper. You or a school-age child can then write their favorite things about Christmas on their ornaments before gluing them onto the tree.

Host Tip
Make as many trees as the kids want… maybe enough for them each to take one home. Remember to date the trees. It's a great keepsake to display year after year.

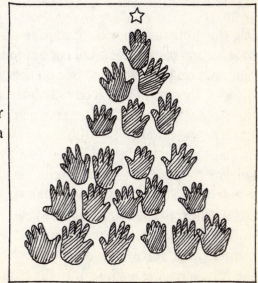

Past and Future

Kwanzaa is a holiday to remind African Americans of their important past and promising future. Here's a fun game that will have children happily moving backward and forward.

What You'll Need	All Ages	Babies	Toddlers	Preschoolers	School-Age Children
Plastic cups	🖐				
Pencils	🖐				
Red, black, and green construction paper	🖐				
Child-safe scissors	🖐				
Silver marker	🖐				
Basket	🖐				

Help the group use the plastic cups to trace circles on the construction paper. Trace and cut out four circles on the red paper, two on the black, and two on the green (see Did You Know? at the end of this activity to learn more about the colors of Kwanzaa). With a marker, you or a school-age child can write the number 1 on the red circles, the number 2 on the black circles, and the number 3 on the green circles. Write the word *forward* on two red circles, one black circle, and one green circle. Then write the word *backward* on the remaining circles. Place all the circles in a basket.

Next, designate a starting point and a finishing point in your play area. Have the kids stand at the starting point and take turns drawing a circle from the basket with eyes closed.

The child then reads the card to determine how many steps to take forward or backward. The game ends when a child reaches the finishing point.

Babies

A baby can play this game, too, with your help. Babies who can grasp objects can draw a circle from the basket. For babies who are showing signs of standing or walking, help them step forward or backward as their cards dictate. If not, the baby will enjoy the movement while being in your arms and close to the rest of the playmates.

Toddlers

This game is a great opportunity to teach toddlers about colors and numbers. When they draw a circle, ask them to first identify its color. Then help them identify the number of steps to take and in what direction. Be sure to count with the toddlers.

Preschoolers and School-Age Children

To emphasize the idea of the past and future, encourage older children to make a wish for the future when they move forward and remember a proud moment from the past when they move backward. For example, when a preschooler draws a circle that has her move forward, she may say, "I wish to learn to ride my bike in the future." When a school-age child draws a circle that has him move backward, he may say, "I'm proud I've learned to ice-skate."

Host Tip
To teach children about the history of Kwanzaa, we recommend reading *K Is for Kwanzaa* by Juwanda G. Ford and *My First Kwanzaa* by Karen Katz.

Did You Know?
The three Kwanzaa colors are green, red, and black: Green represents the color of Africa and also represents hope for the future and continued prosperity. Red represents the color of blood shed by African ancestors who helped African Americans get to the present time. And black represents the color of the African race.

Kwanzaa Corn

Corn is an important symbol in the celebration of Kwanzaa tradition. With this activity, children will make ears of corn that can decorate a table!

What You'll Need	All Ages	Babies	Toddlers	Preschoolers	School-Age Children
Pencils	✋				
Child-safe scissors	✋				
Yellow and green construction paper	✋				
Black paint and shallow bowls			✋	✋	✋
Glue sticks	✋				
Ink pad		✋			
Sponge			✋		
Yarn			✋	✋	✋
Wet wipes		✋			

With older children's help, draw and cut an oval (about nine inches long and three inches wide) for each child from yellow construction paper. Then have each child paint "kernels" so the oval looks like an ear of corn. While the paint dries, help older children cut V shapes from green construction paper to look like husks, then glue them onto the ears when the paint is dry. Display the ears of corn in a basket on your dining-room or kitchen table during the seven days of Kwanzaa (December 26–January 1).

Babies

Babies can help you make ears of corn. To make the "kernels," press one of their thumbs onto an ink pad, then press it all over the ear of corn. For fun, make up a silly song while you work, like "One little, two little, three little kernels!" Have wet wipes handy for cleanup.

Toddlers

Toddlers can sponge paint "kernels" on their ears of corn. From a sponge, cut a square small enough for them to hold (but not small enough to be a choking hazard). Place a shallow bowl with black paint near them and show them how to dip the sponge into the paint then press it lightly onto the ear of corn. Encourage them to sponge paint the entire ear.

Preschoolers and School-Age Children

Show preschoolers and school-age children how to use yarn and paint to create kernels: Have them set their ears of corn horizontally in front of them. Help them cut a piece of yarn that's as long as the ear, then dip it into a shallow bowl of black paint. Show them how to lay the yarn horizontally on the ear, then lift it up so a black line appears across the shape. Have them dip the yarn again and press it about a half inch above or below the line. Repeat this step until the entire shape has horizontal lines at half-inch intervals. Then encourage them to dip the yarn and lay it vertically on the ear of corn, repeating this process so the entire length of the shape has vertical lines at half-inch intervals. The result will be a grid that looks like kernels on an ear of corn.

Feel-Good New Year's Fortunes

Use this variation of an ancient Chinese tradition to look toward a bright future for children on New Year's Day!

What You'll Need	All Ages	Babies	Toddlers	Preschoolers	School-Age Children
Fortunetelling items (see below)	🖐				
Index cards	🖐				
Pencil	🖐				
Scarf or blindfold				🖐	🖐

Before calling children together for the game, gather a number of various household items. For each item, write a symbolic "fortune" on an index card. Here are some examples of potential items and their possible fortunes:

- **Pencil:** *For a future writer or storyteller who has a vivid imagination and loves to share ideas*
- **Book:** *For a future scholar, teacher, or historian who is curious and loves to help others*
- **Spoon:** *For a future chef, baker, or musician who is creative, brave, and self-assured*
- **Paintbrush:** *For a future artist who appreciates the beauty in everything*

Keep each child's interests in mind as you select items. For instance, if one of the toddlers is fascinated with firefighters, add a fire truck and write, "For a future firefighter who is brave, strong, and helpful."

When you finish the cards, fold them in half and place them under each corresponding item. Then call in the children. Don't tell them what each item represents, but have them take turns picking an item. A baby and toddler can motion toward or point to their items, but you may choose to blindfold preschoolers and school-age children to heighten the mystery. When everyone has an object, you or a school-age child can read the cards to reveal the fortunes. If you like, replace the items on the table and play again. Or have children find new items and come up with their own predictions for each one.

Host Tip

Don't underestimate the power of suggestive messages. Need a child to remember to feed the dog? Put out the dog's food bowl with a fortune of "For a wonderful caregiver to all creatures... including your own dog!"

Groundhog Day Silhouettes

Groundhog Day is a traditional yet quirky way to predict the arrival of spring. Kids can celebrate the holiday with this fun shadow activity!

What You'll Need	All Ages	Babies	Toddlers	Preschoolers	School-Age Children
Flashlight	✋				
Black paper	✋				
Tape	✋				
Chalk	✋				
Child-safe scissors	✋				

Have each child take a turn standing in profile in front of a flashlight beam and casting a shadow onto a sheet of black paper taped to the wall. Make sure each sheet is level with the top of each child's head. Use chalk to trace around the shadow, then cut out the silhouette for a wonderful display!

Babies

Try sitting a baby in her highchair or ExerSaucer to trace her shadow. To keep her in profile, encourage her playmates to stand in front of her and make funny faces, sing, and call out her name. Don't worry if she moves around, though—close enough is good enough! Another way to get a great silhouette of a baby is to lay her on the paper and trace around her body.

Toddlers

Toddlers may also have trouble sitting still while you trace their shadow. To help keep them still and amused, ask an older child to read the toddler's favorite book out loud while standing in front of him. When his silhouette is finished, ask them to point out his nose, mouth, chin, and other features.

Preschoolers

At this age, preschoolers will not only sit still for their turn, but they'll also help with the activity. They can cut out their own silhouettes with child-safe scissors. They may also want to hold the flashlight steady as their playmates' silhouettes are drawn. After everyone's silhouette is finished, see if the preschoolers can identify each one. Ask them how they came to their conclusions.

School-Age Children

School-age children can help a lot with this activity. They can tape the paper to the wall, hold the flashlight, and help cut out the silhouettes. They can even trace their playmates' shadows. If you like, ask them to write their wishes for the upcoming spring on the back of their silhouette. Talk about what they can do to make them come true!

Host Tip

While you trace their shadows, explain the Groundhog Day legend to the children: If the groundhog sees its shadow, expect six more weeks of winter. If it doesn't, expect an early spring. For additional fun, use a paper lunch bag as a groundhog and have the creature pop out from under a blanket.

You're in My Heart

Show some love with kids by creating a colorful clay heart together!

What You'll Need	All Ages	Babies	Toddlers	Preschoolers	School-Age Children
Homemade clay (see recipe below)	🖐				
Baking sheet	🖐				
Cooking spray	🖐				
Zip-close plastic bag		🖐			
Marker	🖐				
Butter knife	🖐				
Pencil	🖐				
Yarn	🖐				

Children can help make the clay. Then have kids work together to flatten the red clay on a greased baking sheet so the clay is one to two inches thick. Draw a large heart on the clay with a marker, then cut out the heart shape with a butter knife. Next, the kids can decorate the heart by forming small letters, shapes, or designs with the purple clay and pressing them gently onto the surface of the heart. Tell them this represents how each of them is in the gift receiver's heart!

When they're done, make a hole at the top of the heart with a pencil so you can loop a string through it later for displaying. Bake the heart for thirty to forty minutes at 300°F until the exterior of the dough has formed a crust. When finished, you'll have a decorative heart to display!

Babies

While the other children work on the activity, give the baby a zip-close plastic bag of clay to hold and squeeze. For babies younger than six months, guide their hands to help them explore a piece of clay. Press their fingers into it, but make sure they don't place it in their mouth. You may even want to press babies' fingers into the heart so they can add their own "decoration."

Toddlers

Toddlers will love to pound, tear, and push the clay, which will strengthen their hand muscles. Help them decide what purple designs to add to the heart, then show them how to press them in gently.

Preschoolers

When making the clay, include preschoolers as much as possible. Measuring the ingredients, pouring the liquids, and stirring the dough are great ways for them to learn early math skills and how to follow directions.

School-Age Children

Let school-age children play a large role in preparing the clay, and perhaps let them cut the heart shapes with the butter knife. Once the heart is done, they may also want to make their own hearts or other shapes using the leftover clay. Perhaps they will want to enlist their playmates' help.

Homemade Clay
1½ cups of salt
4 cups of flour
1½ cups of water
Red and blue food coloring

Mix the salt and flour with a spoon in a bowl. Add water gradually. When dough forms, knead it well, adding water if it's too crumbly and flour if it's too sticky. It should be firm. Divide the clay into two bowls. Mix in red food coloring to one bowl. Mix in blue and red food coloring (to make purple) to the other bowl.

At the End of a Rainbow

For Saint Patrick's Day, make a rainbow windsock complete with a trail of dazzling gold coins!

What You'll Need	All Ages	Babies	Toddlers	Preschoolers	School-Age Children
Child-safe scissors	🖐				
Thin cardboard	🖐				
Yellow paint, yellow crayons, and yellow tissue paper and glue	🖐				
Construction paper in rainbow colors	🖐				
Stapler	🖐				
Hole punch	🖐				
Yarn	🖐				
Paintbrushes		🖐	🖐		
Green paint		🖐			
Wet wipes		🖐			

Cut several circles, each about two inches in diameter, from thin cardboard. Give each child some cardboard circles to decorate with yellow paint, yellow crayons, or yellow tissue paper and glue. Set these gold coins aside when finished.

To make each windsock, roll a sheet of green construction paper lengthwise to create a tube. Staple the edges together to hold the tube's shape. You and any older children can then cut one-inch-wide strips from construction paper in rainbow colors. Staple one end of each strip to the tube so the colorful strips dangle from the bottom. Next, punch a hole at the bottom of each strip and at the top of each coin. Using yarn, tie each coin to a strip. Lastly, punch a hole at the top of each tube and string it with yarn so each child can display the windsock outside or inside their homes.

Babies

Give babies cardboard coins to hold and examine. If you like, help them create shamrock designs on the coins: Fold their hands into fists, then paint the pinky-side edge of their hands green. Press their hands onto the coin three times to create a three-leaf clover shape. Use wet wipes to clean their hands when you're done.

Toddlers

When toddlers are decorating their coins, help them use paintbrushes to spread glue onto the coins. They can then press pieces of yellow tissue paper onto the glue.

Preschoolers

Preschoolers can give their coins a textured look. Have them dunk a two-inch length of yarn in the yellow paint. They can coil the yarn on top of the coin in a squiggly spiral, then press the yarn to release the paint. Encourage them to repeat this process until they have covered their coins in paint.

School-Age Children

As the group works on the windsock, challenge any school-age children with a few mathematical questions using the coins.

For example, ask, "If you have ten coins, your friend took three away, and then your other friend gave you two, how many would you have?" They can use the coins to visually figure out the answers.

Did You Know?
Gold coins are one of the oldest forms of money, dating back to 560 BCE.

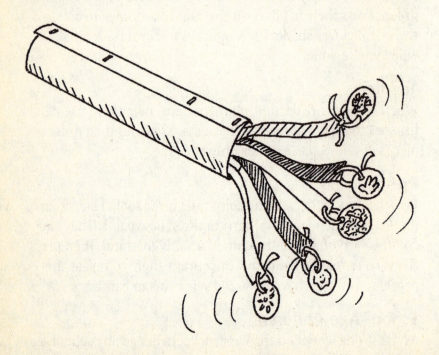

Leprechaun Race

Search for homemade gold coins in a game that will get kids moving.

What You'll Need	All Ages	Babies	Toddlers	Preschoolers	School-Age Children
Large paper bag or box	🖐				
Yellow construction paper	🖐				
Child-safe scissors	🖐				
Marker	🖐				
Construction paper				🖐	

To prepare for this activity, find a large paper bag or box to serve as the "pot." Then make two or three gold "coins" for each child by cutting circles about three inches in diameter from yellow construction paper. On the back of each coin, write simple instructions children can do. For example:

- *Point to your belly.*
- *Clap your hands.*
- *Tap your ears.*
- *Turn around.*
- *Reach for the sky.*
- *Wave your hands.*
- *Shake your neighbor's hand.*
- *Smile and stand still like a statue.*
- *Pretend to dig for gold.*

While the children wait, hide the coins in a room, making sure to stash some in places younger kids can find. When you're done, tell the group to find as many coins as they can and put them into the pot. When they have found all the coins, have each child take a turn picking a coin from the pot. As you or an older child reads the back of the coin, encourage everyone to follow the instructions!

Babies

Accompany babies during the coin hunt. If they are mobile, direct them toward a coin within their reach. They can retrieve it and drop it into the pot. Also help them follow the instructions on the coins, if needed. But they may surprise you by watching the others and following some instructions themselves, like finding their belly or reaching up high!

Toddlers

Toddlers will gain confidence as they find coins. If they need a little direction, point them toward the general location by saying things such as, "Look near the toy box." Finding the coins, putting them into the pot, and following the instructions will strengthen a toddler's abilities to listen and concentrate. Give them lots of encouragement as they complete these tasks.

Preschoolers

Preschoolers will search enthusiastically for coins around the room. To challenge them in a different way, however, give them special instructions: Before they can drop a coin in the pot, they must turn it over and identify three letters from the sentence. Once they call the letters out loud, they can drop the coin and return to the search.

School-Age Children

School-age children may enjoy reading the instructions on each coin out loud to the group. If you like, you can read the instructions and tell school-age children that they have a special rule: They can follow the instructions only if they first hear the phrase, "The leprechaun says…" This activity will encourage careful listening, especially because their playmates will be following the instructions regardless of the preface!

Index

434